WORKBOOK TO ACCOMPANY
Clinical Application
of Mechanical Ventilation

WORKBOOK TO ACCOMPANY
Clinical Application of Mechanical Ventilation

FOURTH EDITION

David W. Chang

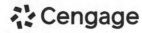

Australia • Brazil • Canada • Mexico • Singapore • United Kingdom • United States

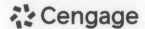

Workbook to Accompany Clinical Application of Mechanical Ventilation, Fourth Edition
David W. Chang

Vice President, Careers & Computing: Dave Garza

Publisher, Health Care: Stephen Helba

Associate Acquisitions Editor: Christina Gifford

Director, Development—Careers & Computing: Marah Bellegarde

Product Development Manager, Careers: Juliet Steiner

Associate Product Manager: Meghan E. Orvis

Editorial Assistant: Cassie Cloutier

Executive Brand Manager: Wendy Mapstone

Market Development Manager: Jonathan Sheehan

Senior Production Director: Wendy A. Troeger

Production Manager: Andrew Crouth

Senior Content Project Manager: Kara A. DiCaterino

Senior Art Director: David Arsenault

Cover Image:
© Icons Jewelry/www.shutterstock.com
© Sebastian Kaulitzki/www.shutterstock.com

For product information and technology assistance, contact us at
Cengage Customer & Sales Support, 1-800-354-9706 or support.cengage.com.

For permission to use material from this text or product, submit all requests online at **www.copyright.com.**

ISBN-13: 978-1-111-53967-2
ISBN-10: 1-111-53967-7

Cengage
200 Pier 4 Boulevard
Boston, MA 02210
USA

Cengage is a leading provider of customized learning solutions with employees residing in nearly 40 different countries and sales in more than 125 countries around the world. Find your local representative at: **www.cengage.com.**

To learn more about Cengage platforms and services, register or access your online learning solution, or purchase materials for your course, visit **www.cengage.com.**

Printed in the United States of America
Print Number: 09   Print Year: 2023

Contents

Contents

Preface

This workbook reinforces the essential concepts presented in *Clinical Application of Mechanical Ventilation*, Fourth Edition, giving learners the opportunity to practice with questions written in the NRBC format. With a concise, easy-to-read approach, this workbook integrates the essential concepts of respiratory physiology with the clinical application of mechanical ventilation. The questions correspond to the core book reinforcing key topics. While questions are written in the NRBC format they also cover all NRBC content areas.

Content areas covered include:

- Airway management and weaning criteria
- Pharmacology for mechanical ventilation
- Special procedures in mechanical ventilation, chest tubes and placement, proportional pressure support, airway management, and ventilator waveform analysis

New to the Fourth Edition

- All questions have been updated to reflect the new Fourth Edition of *Clinical Applications of Mechanical Ventilation*.
- Chapter 15: Critical Care Issues in Mechanical Ventilation is a new chapter corresponding to the new content in the core textbook.
- Updated coverage of mechanical ventilation in nontraditional settings goes beyond home mechanical ventilation.

CHAPTER 1

Principles of Mechanical Ventilation

INTRODUCTION

1. Mechanical ventilation is commonly used to manage all of the following conditions *except*:

    A. correction of severe hypoxemia.

    B. correction of acute carbon dioxide retention.

    C. support of ventilatory failure.

    D. compensation of acid-base imbalance.

2. Mechanical ventilation is usually *not* indicated in conditions such as:

    A. ventilatory failure.

    B. metabolic acidosis.

    C. chest trauma.

    D. postoperative recovery.

3. One of the most frequent uses of mechanical ventilation is for the management of _____ (preoperative, postoperative) patients _____ (before receiving, recovering from) anesthesia and medications.

4. Select the six pathophysiologic factors or changes below that is most likely an indication for mechanical ventilation.

    (1) _____ (Apnea, Tachypnea)

    (2) _____ (Acute respiratory alkalosis, Impending respiratory arrest)

    (3) _____ (COPD, Acute exacerbation of COPD)

    (4) _____ (Chronic bronchitis, Acute severe asthma)

    (5) _____ (Neuromuscular disease, Hypertension)

    (6) _____ (Flail chest, Tension pneumothorax)

5. Patients who require mechanical ventilation commonly have clinical signs of ventilatory failure, oxygenation failure, or both. _____ (TRUE/FALSE)

AIRWAY RESISTANCE

6. Airway resistance is the degree of _____ obstruction in the airways.

7. Describe the factors that may affect the airway resistance during mechanical ventilation.

   _____

   _____

8. Airflow obstruction may be caused by all of the following changes *except*:

   A. increased lung compliance.

   B. retained secretions in the airways.

   C. neoplasm of the bronchial muscle structure.

   D. tumors compressing the airway.

9. When the radius of an airway decreases by half (50%) of its original size, the driving pressure needed to maintain the same airflow must increase by a factor of _____ (2-fold, 16-fold, 100-fold).

10 to 12. Match the type of airflow obstruction with the clinical conditions that may increase a patient's airway resistance.

TYPE	CLINICAL CONDITIONS
10. _____ COPD	A. Condensation in ventilator circuit
11. _____ Mechanical obstruction	B. Epiglottitis
12. _____ Infection	C. Chronic asthma

13. During mechanical ventilation, one of the strategies to reduce the airflow resistance is to:

    A. lengthen the endotracheal tube.

    B. use the smallest endotracheal tube possible.

    C. remove the secretions in the endotracheal tube.

    D. add water to the ventilator circuit.

14. Airway resistance and work of breathing are _____ (directly, inversely) related. In other words, the work of breathing is _____ (increased, decreased) in conditions of high airway resistance.

15. If the work of breathing cannot keep pace with the increase of airway resistance, the airflow will _____ (increase, decrease).

16. In order to compensate or accommodate for the increase in airflow resistance, patients with chronic airway obstruction typically use a breathing pattern that is _____ (deep and slow, shallow and fast).

17. Under respiratory stress or severe hypoxia, patients with restrictive lung disease use a breathing pattern that is _____ (deep and slow, shallow and fast) since reduced lung compliance is the primary disturbance for these patients.

18. When an abnormally high airway resistance is sustained over a long time, all of the following may occur with the *exception* of:

    A. fatigue of the respiratory muscles.

    B. metabolic alkalosis.

    C. ventilatory failure.

    D. oxygenation failure.

19. On the pressure-volume loop, increase in bowing of the inspiratory limb suggests:

    A. excessive inspiratory flow.

    B. insufficient inspiratory flow.

    C. increased lung compliance.

    D. decreased lung compliance.

LUNG COMPLIANCE

20. Given: Corrected V_T 600 mL, peak inspiratory pressure 45 cm H_2O, plateau pressure 35 cm H_2O, PEEP 5 cm H_2O. Calculate the static compliance (C_{ST}) and dynamic compliance (C_{DYN}).

    A. C_{ST} = 13 mL/cm H_2O, C_{DYN} = 17 mL/cm H_2O

    B. C_{ST} = 15 mL/cm H_2O, C_{DYN} = 20 mL/cm H_2O

    C. C_{ST} = 17 mL/cm H_2O, C_{DYN} = 13 mL/cm H_2O

    D. C_{ST} = 20 mL/cm H_2O, C_{DYN} = 15 mL/cm H_2O

21. Since the peak inspiratory pressure is _____ (equal to, higher than, lower than) the plateau pressure, which of the following statements is true concerning the calculated compliance values?

    A. The dynamic compliance is the same as the static compliance.

    B. The dynamic compliance is greater than the static compliance.

    C. The dynamic compliance is lower than the static compliance.

    D. Insufficient information to provide answer.

22. Extreme _____ (high, low) compliance makes lung expansion difficult, whereas extreme _____ (high, low) compliance leads to poor elastic recoil of the lung tissues, incomplete exhalation, and CO_2 retention.

23. _____ (High, Low) compliance or _____ (high, low) elastance means that the volume change is small per unit pressure change. Under this condition, the lungs are considered "stiff" or _____ (compliant, noncompliant).

24. Compliance and work of breathing are _____ (directly, inversely) related. In other words, the work of breathing is _____ (increased, decreased) in conditions of *low* compliance.

25. If the work of breathing cannot keep pace with the continuing decrease in compliance, the tidal volume will _____ (increase, decrease) as a result.

26. When an abnormally *low* compliance is sustained over a long time, all of the following may occur with the exception of:

    A. oxygenation failure.

    B. ventilatory failure.

    C. respiratory muscle fatigue.

    D. acute renal failure.

27. Mr. Jones, a patient diagnosed with adult respiratory distress syndrome, has a static compliance of 15 mL/cm H_2O (normal is 40 to 60 mL/cm H_2O). Based on the compliance value, which of the following assumptions is most likely true?

    A. The patient's functional residual capacity is increased.

    B. The elastic recoil of the lungs is decreased.

    C. The patient may have an obstructive lung defect.

    D. The patient's work of breathing is increased.

28. When the compliance value is extremely high (e.g., emphysema), exhalation is often _____ (improved, incomplete) due to a(n) _____ (increase, decrease) of lung elastic recoil during exhalation.

29. High compliance measurement may be related to conditions of _____ (increased, decreased) functional residual capacity, _____ (obstructive, restrictive) lung defect, airflow obstruction, incomplete exhalation, air trapping, and poor gas exchange.

30. In general, the static compliance is affected by changes in the _____ (airway, lung parenchyma). An example of this condition is _____ (bronchospasm, pneumonia, mucus plug).

31. Airway obstruction primarily leads to changes in the _____ (static, dynamic) compliance.

32. Since static compliance is measured when there is _____ (high, little or no) airflow, airway resistance _____ (is, is not) a determining factor of the static compliance measurement.

33. Static compliance reflects the _____ (elastic, nonelastic) properties of the lung and chest wall, and it is known as the _____ (elastic, nonelastic) resistance.

34. Since dynamic compliance is measured when airflow is _____ (present, absent), airway resistance _____ (is, is not) a determining factor of the dynamic compliance measurement.

35. Dynamic compliance is calculated by dividing the tidal volume by the _____ (peak inspiratory pressure, plateau pressure). This pressure is required to overcome the _____ (airflow resistance, compliance, airflow resistance and compliance).

36. In general, conditions causing changes in the static compliance invoke _____ (similar, different) changes in the dynamic compliance. For example, atelectasis _____ (increases, decreases) the _____ (static, dynamic, static and dynamic) compliance measurements.

37. In conditions where the lung compliance is decreased, the:

    A. peak inspiratory pressure is increased.

    B. plateau pressure is decreased.

    C. peak inspiratory pressure and plateau pressure are both increased.

    D. peak inspiratory pressure and plateau pressure are both decreased.

38. In conditions where the lung compliance is decreased, the:

    A. static compliance is increased.

    B. dynamic compliance is decreased.

    C. static compliance and dynamic compliance are both increased.

    D. static compliance and dynamic compliance are both decreased.

39. In conditions where the airflow resistance is increased, the:

    A. peak inspiratory pressure is decreased.

    B. plateau pressure is increased.

    C. peak inspiratory pressure is increased while the plateau pressure remains the same.

    D. peak inspiratory pressure is decreased while the plateau pressure remains the same.

40. In conditions where the airflow resistance is increased, the:

    A. static compliance is increased.

    B. dynamic compliance is increased.

    C. dynamic compliance is decreased while the static compliance remains the same.

    D. static compliance is decreased while the dynamic compliance remains the same.

41. Shifting of the pressure-volume loop toward the pressure axis indicates a(n):

    A. increase in airflow resistance.

    B. decrease in airflow resistance.

    C. increase in lung compliance.

    D. decrease in lung compliance.

42. In nonintubated subjects, the normal dynamic compliance is between _____ (1 and 3; 30 and 40; 300 and 400) mL/cm H_2O, and the normal static compliance is between _____ (3 and 6; 40 and 60; 500 and 600) mL/cm H_2O.

DEADSPACE VENTILATION

43. Deadspace ventilation is defined as wasted ventilation or a condition in which _____ (ventilation, pulmonary blood flow) is in excess of _____ (ventilation, pulmonary blood flow).

44. The anatomic deadspace of a 140-lb patient may be estimated to be _____ (70, 100, 140, 180) mL.

45. Decrease in tidal volume leads to a _____ (higher, lower) anatomic deadspace to tidal volume (V_D/V_T) ratio.

46. Alveolar deadspace ventilation occurs when the ventilated alveoli are _____ (overly, not adequately) perfused by the pulmonary circulation.

47. Alveolar deadspace ventilation may be caused by all of the following conditions *except*:

    A. pulmonary vasoconstriction.

    B. congestive heart failure.

    C. blood loss.

    D. atelectasis.

48. Physiologic deadspace is the _____ (sum, difference, product) of anatomic and alveolar deadspace volumes. Under normal conditions, the physiologic deadspace is about the same as the _____ (anatomic, alveolar) deadspace.

49. Measurement of the physiologic deadspace to tidal volume ratio (V_D/V_T) requires a(n):

    A. arterial blood gas sample.

    B. mixed expired gas sample.

    C. pulmonary artery blood gas sample.

    D. arterial and mixed expired gas samples.

50. The physiologic deadspace to tidal volume ratio (V_D/V_T) is calculated by:

    A. $V_D/V_T = (PaCO_2 - P_ECO_2)$.

    B. $V_D/V_T = (PaCO_2 - P_ECO_2)/PaCO_2$.

    C. $V_D/V_T = (PaCO_2 - P_ECO_2)/PaCO_2$.

    D. $V_D/V_T = (PaCO_2 - P_ECO_2)/PaCO_2$.

51. V_D/V_T of less than 60% reflects _____ (normal, abnormal) ventilatory function on successful weaning from mechanical ventilation.

52. Prolonged and excessive deadspace ventilation causes inefficient ventilation, muscle fatigue, ventilatory and oxygenation failure. _____ (TRUE/FALSE)

VENTILATORY FAILURE

53. Define ventilatory failure.

    _____

    _____

54. The key feature of ventilatory failure is _____ (hypercapnia, hypocapnia) or a significant _____ (increase, decrease) of arterial PCO_2.

55. Respiratory acidosis occurs when carbon dioxide _____ (removal, production) exceeds its _____ (removal, production).

56 to 60. Match the mechanisms leading to the development of ventilatory failure with the typical findings. Use each answer only *once*.

MECHANISM	CLINICAL FINDING
56. _____ Hypoventilation	A. $Q_s/Q_T > 20\%$ (>30% in critical shunt)
57. _____ Persistent V/Q mismatch	B. Low barometric pressure as in high altitude
58. _____ Persistent intrapulmonary shunt	C. Gas diffusion rate < 75% of predicted normal
59. _____ Persistent diffusion defect	D. $PaCO_2$ >45 mm Hg (>50 mm Hg for patients with COPD)
60. _____ Persistent reduction of P_IO_2	E. Hypoxemia that responds well to oxygen therapy

61. Which of the following conditions is *least* likely a cause of alveolar hypoventilation?

    A. Metabolic acidosis

    B. Depression of breathing centers

    C. Neuromuscular disease

    D. Airway obstruction

62. In reviewing a patient's chart, the admitting note states that the patient was *hypoventilating* on arrival at the emergency department. This assessment is based on an increase of the patient's _____ (spontaneous tidal volume, spontaneous respiratory frequency, pulse oximetry saturation, arterial carbon dioxide tension).

63. Based on the equation: $V_A = V_T - V_D$, a patient's alveolar volume can be increased by:

    A. increasing the tidal volume (V_T).

    B. increasing the deadspace volume (V_D).

    C. decreasing the tidal volume (V_T).

    D. decreasing the tidal volume (V_T) and deadspace volume (V_D).

64. Since minute alveolar ventilation ($\dot{V}_A$) is a function of the tidal volume (V_T), deadspace volume (V_D), and respiratory frequency (f) as shown in the equation: $\dot{V}_A = (V_T - \dot{V}_D) \times f$, hypoventilation may be corrected by:

    A. decreasing the V_T.

    B. decreasing the f.

    C. increasing the f.

    D. increasing the V_D.

65. A physician wants to monitor Mr. Smith's *ventilatory* status. The therapist should measure the patient's _____ (pH, PaO_2, $PaCO_2$, respiratory frequency) on an as-needed basis.

66. Based on the equation: $\dot{V}_A = \dot{V}CO_2/PaCO_2$, an increase of carbon dioxide production ($\dot{V}CO_2$) would cause a(n) _____ (increase, decrease) of the arterial carbon dioxide tension ($PaCO_2$) level. (Assume the $\dot{V}_A$ remains unchanged.)

67. Define V/Q mismatch.

   _____

   _____

68. A _____ (high, low) V/Q ratio may be seen in pulmonary embolism where the pulmonary _____ (ventilation, perfusion) is reduced.

69. In airway obstruction, pulmonary _____ (ventilation, perfusion) is reduced and it leads to a _____ (high, low) V/Q ratio.

70. Hypoxemia caused by mild or simple V/Q mismatch is generally _____ (readily, not) reversible by oxygen therapy alone.

71. Define intrapulmonary shunting.

   _____

   _____

72. Define refractory hypoxemia.

   _____

   _____

73. Since shunted pulmonary blood flow _____ (does, does not) come in contact with ventilated and oxygenated alveoli, oxygen therapy alone is usually an _____ (effective, ineffective) treatment for shunting.

74. A hemodynamic study reveals that Ms. Jamison's shunt percent is 35%. This may be interpreted as a _____ (normal, mild, significant, critical and severe) intrapulmonary shunt.

75. The *estimated* physiologic shunt equation for a *critically ill* patient is:

   A. Estimated $Q_S/Q_T = (CcO_2 - CaO_2)/[2 + (CcO_2 - CaO_2)]$.

   B. Estimated $Q_S/Q_T = (CcO_2 - CaO_2)/[3.5 + (CcO_2 - CaO_2)]$.

   C. Estimated $Q_S/Q_T = (CcO_2 - CaO_2)/[5 + (CcO_2 - CaO_2)]$.

   D. Estimated $Q_S/Q_T = (CcO_2 - CaO_2)/[16 + (CcO_2 - CaO_2)]$.

76. As shown below, the *classic* physiologic shunt equation requires measurement of _____ (one, two, three) blood sample(s).

   Classic $Q_S/Q_T = (CcO_2 - CaO_2)/(CcO_2 - CvO_2)$.

77 to 80. Match the causes of decreased diffusion rate with the clinical conditions. Use each answer *once*.

TYPE OF DIFFUSION PROBLEM	CLINICAL CONDITIONS
77. _____ Decrease of pressure gradient	A. Pulmonary edema, retained secretions
78. _____ Thickening of A-c membrane	B. Tachycardia
79. _____ Decreased surface area of lungs	C. Emphysema, pulmonary fibrosis
80. _____ Insufficient time for gas diffusion	D. High altitude, fire combustion

OXYGENATION FAILURE

81. Oxygenation failure is defined as severe _____ (hyperventilation, hypoventilation, hypoxemia) that does not respond to moderate-to-high levels of _____ (mechanical ventilation, supplemental oxygen).

82. Since arterial PO_2 (PaO_2) measures the amount of oxygen _____ (dissolved in the plasma, combined with hemoglobin), it _____ (does, does not) accurately reflect the oxygenation status of patients with dysfunctional hemoglobins (e.g., carbon monoxide poisoning).

83. Differentiate hypoxemia and hypoxia.

_____

_____

84. Hypoxia can occur with a PaO_2 of 85 mm Hg. _____ (TRUE/FALSE)

85. The important clinical signs of oxygenation failure and hypoxia include all of the following *except*:

    A. hypothermia.

    B. dyspnea.

    C. tachypnea.

    D. tachycardia.

CLINICAL CONDITIONS LEADING TO MECHANICAL VENTILATION

86. Depressed respiratory drive is one of the indications for mechanical ventilation. Which of the following conditions is *least* likely to affect a patient's normal respiratory drive?

    A. Spinal cord injury at cervical-2 (C-2) level

    B. Drug overdose

    C. Chest trauma

    D. Head injury

87. Excessive ventilatory workload is one of the indications for mechanical ventilation. Which of the following conditions is *least* likely to increase a patient's ventilatory workload?

   A. Airflow obstruction

   B. Deadspace ventilation

   C. Decreased compliance

   D. Drug overdose

88. Failure of the ventilatory pump is one of the indications for mechanical ventilation. Which of the following conditions does *not* normally lead to failure of the ventilatory pump?

   A. Hyperkalemia

   B. Hypothermia

   C. Flail chest

   D. Fatigue of respiratory muscles

Effects of Positive Pressure Ventilation

PULMONARY CONSIDERATIONS

1. During spontaneous ventilation, the diaphragm and other respiratory muscles create gas flow by _____ (increasing, decreasing) the pleural, alveolar, and airway pressures.

2. When the alveolar and airway pressures become _____ (higher than, lower than) the atmospheric pressure, air flows into the lungs.

3. In negative pressure ventilation, the pressures in the airways, alveoli, and pleura are _____ (increased, decreased) during inspiration, whereas in positive pressure ventilation, the same pressures are _____ (increased, decreased).

4. With normal airway resistance and compliance, a higher positive pressure applied to the lungs results in a _____ (larger, smaller) tidal volume.

5. During pressure-controlled ventilation, when the peak inspiratory pressure is reached prematurely, the tidal volume delivered to the patient will be _____ (higher, lower) than normal.

6. All of the following clinical conditions may cause the inspiratory phase to end prematurely *except*:

   A. circuit disconnect.

   B. airway obstruction.

   C. kinking of endotracheal tube.

   D. low lung compliance.

7. _____ is a condition that prevents a ventilator to reach its preset pressure or volume.

   A. Kinking of ventilator circuit

   B. Low lung compliance

   C. High airway resistance

   D. Endotracheal tube cuff leak

8. During pressure-controlled ventilation, the _____ (volume, pressure) is preset and the _____ (volume, pressure) delivered by the ventilator is *variable*.

9. During volume-controlled ventilation, the _____ (volume, pressure) is preset and the _____ (volume, pressure) generated by the ventilator is *variable*.

10. In patients with _____ (compliant, noncompliant) lungs, the effects of positive pressure on the cardiac output is less severe because _____ (more, less) pressure is transmitted from the airways to the lung parenchyma.

CARDIOVASCULAR CONSIDERATIONS

11. Positive pressure ventilation typically _____ (increases, decreases) the mean airway pressure (mPaw) and _____ (increases, decreases) a patient's cardiac output.

12. A mechanically ventilated patient has a calculated mean airway pressure (mPaw) of 40 cm H_2O, and the physician would like to lower it in order to minimize the cardiovascular side effects. The therapist should:

    A. increase the peak inspiratory pressure.

    B. increase the frequency.

    C. decrease the tidal volume.

    D. initiate positive end-expiratory pressure (PEEP).

13. Given: O_2 content × cardiac output = O_2 delivery.

    Since positive pressure ventilation commonly leads to a(n) _____ (increase, decrease) of the cardiac output, the oxygen delivery is likely to be _____ (increased, reduced) as a result. (Assume the O_2 content remains unchanged.)

14. In patients with cardiopulmonary disease or compromised cardiovascular reserve, positive pressure ventilation may cause the blood pressure measurements to _____ (increase, decrease).

15. Due to the thoracic pump mechanism, an increase of tidal volume causes a decrease of venous return to the left ventricle in _____ (hypertensive, hypotensive) patients.

16. During spontaneous inspiration, a transient decrease of arterial blood pressure is called _____ (pulsus paradoxus, reverse pulsus paradoxus).

17. A significant reverse pulsus paradoxus (increase of systolic pressure >15 mm Hg) during positive pressure ventilation is a sensitive indicator of _____ (hypervolemia, hypovolemia).

HEMODYNAMIC CONSIDERATIONS

18. Positive pressure ventilation causes a(n) _____ (increase, decrease) of the intrathoracic pressure and compression of the pulmonary blood vessels. This condition causes an overall _____ (increase, decrease) in ventricular output, stroke volume, and pressure readings.

19. The severity of hemodynamic changes during positive pressure ventilation is affected by the airway pressures, lung volume, and compliance characteristics of the patient. _____ (TRUE/ FALSE)

20. The intrathoracic pressure is _____ (increased, decreased) during mechanical ventilation because the positive pressure applied to the lungs causes _____ (expansion, compression) of the lung parenchyma against the chest wall.

21. During the *inspiratory* phase of positive pressure ventilation, a fraction of the _____ (systemic, pulmonary) blood volume is shifted to the _____ (systemic, pulmonary) circulation. This causes a transient _____ (increase, decrease) of the pulmonary blood volume.

22. A higher intrathoracic pressure _____ (enhances, impedes) the systemic blood return to the right ventricle. This results in a _____ (higher, lower) venous return and a higher central venous pressure (CVP) reading.

23. A lower venous return to the right ventricle leads to a _____ (higher, lower) right ventricular output and a _____ (higher, lower) blood volume in the pulmonary arterial system.

24. Since volume and pressure are two _____ (directly, inversely) related variables, a lower blood volume in the pulmonary arterial system leads to a _____ (higher, lower) pulmonary arterial pressure (PAP) reading.

25. As the left ventricle receives less blood from the pulmonary circulation, the left ventricular output is _____ (increased, unchanged, decreased).

26. In the absence of compensation by increasing the heart rate, decrease of right and left ventricular stroke volumes generally leads to a decreased cardiac output. _____ (TRUE/FALSE)

27. The hemodynamic effects of PEEP are highly variable and dependent on a patient's condition. In general, PEEP causes a(n) _____ (increase, decrease) of the pulmonary artery pressure and the central venous pressure but a(n) _____ (increase, decrease) of the aortic pressure and cardiac output.

28. PEEP leads to a(n) _____ (increase, decrease) of the PAP because PEEP causes significant compression of the pulmonary blood vessels.

29. An increase of PAP causes a higher right ventricular pressure and hinders the blood return from systemic circulation to right heart. This causes backup of blood flow and a(n) _____ (increase, decrease) of pressure in the systemic venous circulation (i.e., central venous pressure).

30. PEEP leads to a _____ (higher, lower) aortic pressure because of a significant increase of the intrathoracic pressure and significant reduction of the left and right ventricular stroke volumes.

31. PEEP leads to a _____ (higher, lower) cardiac output for the same reasons affecting the aortic pressure.

RENAL CONSIDERATIONS

32. When renal perfusion is decreased, filtration and reabsorption become _____ (more, less) efficient. As a result, the urine output is _____ (increased, decreased) as the kidneys try to correct this _____ (hypervolemic, hypovolemic) condition by _____ (releasing, retaining) fluid.

33. For adequate removal of body wastes, the urine output must be above _____ (100 mL, 200 mL, 300 mL, 400 mL) in a 24-hour period. Therefore, a(n) _____ (increased, decreased) urine output is an early sign of renal insufficiency or failure.

34. Inadequate urine output is called _____ and is defined as a urine output of less than _____ mL in 24 hours or less than _____ mL in 8 hours.

35. Other early signs of renal failure include _____ (elevation, reduction) of the serum blood urea nitrogen (BUN) level to _____ (more than, less than) 20 mg/dL; the creatinine level to _____ (more than, less than) 1.5 mg/dL; and a BUN to creatinine ratio greater than _____ (5-to-1, 10-to-1).

36. In addition to elimination of wastes, kidneys are responsible for the regulation of all of the following *except*:

    A. spinal fluid pressure.

    B. drug clearance.

    C. fluid and electrolyte balance.

    D. acid-base balance.

37. During positive pressure ventilation, hypoperfusion of the kidneys may _____ (increase, decrease) the rate of drug clearance leading to a _____ (higher, lower) drug concentration in the circulation.

38. For drugs that rely on renal clearance, the concentration in the circulation may be increased in all of the following conditions with the *exception* of:

    A. decrease of glomerular filtration rate.

    B. decrease of tubular secretion.

    C. increase of renal perfusion.

    D. hypovolemia.

39. In low-cardiac-output situations, the urine and drug concentrations in the urine are _____ (higher, lower) than normal and this may lead to a _____ (higher, lower) reabsorption rate of the drugs back into the circulation.

HEPATIC CONSIDERATIONS

40. The liver is perfused by about 15% of the total cardiac output, and this perfusion rate may be reduced when _____ (oxygen, pressure support, PEEP) is added to positive pressure ventilation.

41. All of the following laboratory measurements may indicate the presence of liver dysfunction with the *exception* of:

    A. prothrombin time >4 sec over control.

    B. hematocrit >40%.

    C. bilirubin level ≥50 mg/L.

    D. albumin level ≤20 g/L.

42. Clearance of lidocaine, meperidine, propranolol, and verapamil relies on adequate liver function and perfusion. When the gastrointestinal (GI) hepatic perfusion is inadequate, use of these drugs may lead to a relatively _____ (higher, lower) drug concentration due to _____ (enhanced, impaired) drug clearance.

ABDOMINAL CONSIDERATIONS

43. Increased intra-abdominal pressure (IAP) may transmit the excessive pressure across the diaphragm to the heart and great vessels. In turn, this leads to _____ (increased, decreased) cardiac output and _____ (increased, decreased) renal perfusion.

44. Use of PEEP at a level greater than _____ (5, 10, 15) cm H_2O in the presence of high IAP (>20 mm Hg) requires caution because of the potentiation of the pressures exerted on the heart and great vessels.

45. Excessive PEEP and IAP may lead to all of the following complications *except*:

    A. increased atelectasis.

    B. impaired gas exchange.

    C. increased V/Q mismatch.

    D. increased functional residual capacity.

GASTROINTESTINAL CONSIDERATIONS

46. GI complications in patients who are being mechanically ventilated include all of the following *except*:

    A. erosive esophagitis.

    B. diarrhea or constipation.

    C. increased bowel sounds.

    D. stress-related mucosal damage.

47. GI complications in mechanically ventilated patients are usually due to decreased GI perfusion and medications commonly administered to these patients. _____ (TRUE/FALSE)

NUTRITIONAL CONSIDERATIONS

48. Nutritional balance is vital in the management of critically ill patients because malnutrition may cause _____ (excessive CO_2 production, muscle fatigue), whereas excessive nutritional support may cause _____ (excessive CO_2 production, muscle fatigue).

49. COPD patients have higher caloric needs because of the increased work of breathing associated with chronic airflow obstruction. _____ (TRUE/FALSE)

50. Fatigue of the respiratory muscles and ventilatory failure are most likely to occur in conditions where the:

   A. airway resistance is low.

   B. chest wall compliance is high.

   C. lung compliance is low.

   D. work of breathing is low.

51. In addition to malnutrition, list four conditions that may lead to respiratory muscle fatigue.

   _____

   _____

   _____

   _____

52. Describe the process of undernutrition leading to a reduction of ventilatory efficiency.

   _____

   _____

   _____

53. The energy requirements for critically ill patients should be computed by using the Harris-Benedict equation and the patient's activity or stress factor during hospitalization. _____ (TRUE/FALSE)

54. _____ (More, Less) nutritional supplementation is needed for ventilator patients who are hypermetabolic or hypercatabolic due to conditions such as infection, trauma, and burns.

55. For patients with CO_2 retention, a _____ (fat-based, glucose-based) parenteral diet supplement is preferred because it provides _____ (more, less) kcal per gram and _____ (higher, lower) CO_2 production.

NEUROLOGIC CONSIDERATIONS

56. In mechanical ventilation, intentional hyperventilation is sometimes used to reduce the _____ (pH, intrapulmonary pressure, intracranial pressure) in patients with head injury.

57. Sustained hyperventilation of less than 24 hours causes respiratory _____ (acidosis, alkalosis) and a(n) _____ (increase, reduction) of cerebral blood flow and intracranial pressure.

58. List three side effects of prolonged (>24 hours) hyperventilation.

   _____

   _____

   _____

59. Hypoventilation and abnormalities in gas exchange can cause all of the following conditions *except*:

A. secondary anemia.

B. respiratory acidosis.

C. hypoxemia.

D. secondary polycythemia.

60. Mr. Kingston, a patient who was weaned from mechanical ventilation 2 days ago, complains of pressure headache, motor disturbances, and ocular abnormalities. While talking with him, he appears to have moderate deterioration in his mental status. These complaints and observation are suggestive of:

A. sustained hyperventilation.

B. neurologic impairment.

C. electrolyte imbalance.

D. oxygen toxicity.

61. _____ (Hypercapnia, Hypocapnia) may cause muscle tremor and ocular abnormalities.

62. Muscle tremor is the result of excessive _____ (stimulation, suppression) of the sympathetic nervous system and catecholamine release from the adrenal medulla.

63. Ocular abnormalities are the result of cerebral _____ (vasodilation, vasoconstriction) and _____ (elevation, depression) of intracranial pressure.

64 to 66. Match the pulmonary conditions with the neurologic changes. Use each answer only *once*.

PULMONARY CONDITIONS	PHYSIOLOGIC CHANGES
64. _____ Hypercapnia (with low pH)	A. Decreased mental and motor functions
65. _____ Hypercapnia (with normal pH)	B. Impaired cerebral metabolism
66. _____ Hypoxemia	C. Increased cerebral blood flow and intracranial pressure

CHAPTER 3

Classification of Mechanical Ventilators

VENTILATOR CLASSIFICATION

1. A classification system for ventilators is used to learn the _____ (waveform, operational, pressure, safety) characteristics of each ventilator.

2. Ventilators may be classified by their:

   A. similarities.

   B. differences.

   C. manufacturers.

   D. A and B only.

VENTILATORY WORK

3. Mechanical ventilators generate gas flow and deliver lung volume by creating a transairway _____ (compliance, volume, pressure) gradient.

4. The tidal volume delivered to the patient by the mechanical ventilator is _____ (directly, inversely) related to the transairway pressure gradient.

5. In order to create sufficient gas flow and adequate lung volume, the patient or ventilator must overcome the opposing force of:

   A. compliance.

   B. resistance.

   C. conductance.

   D. A and B only.

6. _____ (Compliance, Resistance, Elastance, Conductance) is a measurement that describes how much volume (mL) can be delivered by applying one unit of pressure (cm H_2O).

7. Pressure gradient (ΔP) divided by flow represents the _____ (conductance, compliance, resistance, elastance) measurement.

INPUT POWER

8. Pneumatically powered ventilators use _____ (electricity, compressed gas) as an energy source for their operation.

9. Give at least two examples of pneumatically powered ventilators.

    _____

    _____

    _____

10. _____ (Pneumatically, Electrically) powered ventilators may use 120 V 60 Hz alternating current (AC) or 12 V direct current (DC) for a power source.

11. Give at least two examples of electrically powered ventilators.

    _____

    _____

    _____

12. Name two ventilators that are powered by a combination of pneumatic and electric power sources.

    _____

    _____

DRIVE MECHANISM

13. The drive mechanism is the system used by a ventilator to convert the input power to gas flow and tidal volume. _____ (TRUE/FALSE)

14. Name three drive mechanisms for ventilators.

    _____

    _____

    _____

15. Rotary- or linear-driven pistons use one-way valves to compress the gas, generate a _____ (pressure, volume, temperature) gradient, and drive a ventilator.

16. Bellows drive ventilators use a bellows to _____ (clean, divert, filter, compress) the gas for delivery to the patient.

MICROPROCESSOR-CONTROLLED PNEUMATIC DRIVE MECHANISM

17. When a ventilator uses microprocessors to open and close the solenoid valves, the process is called a microprocessor-controlled _____ (piston, bellows, pressure, pneumatic) drive mechanism.

CONTROL CIRCUIT

18. The control circuit is the system that governs or controls the ventilator _____ or output control valve.

19. An open-loop control circuit is one where the desired output is selected and the ventilator achieves the desired output _____ (with additional, without any further) input from the clinician or the ventilator.

20. A closed-loop control circuit is one where the _____ (input, output) is constantly adjusted to match the desired _____ (input, output). This type of control circuit may also be referred to as _____ (servo-, feedback-) controlled.

21. _____ (Mechanical, Pneumatic, Fluidic, Electric, Electronic) control circuits employ simple machines such as levers, pulleys, or cams to control the drive mechanism.

22. _____ (Mechanical, Pneumatic, Fluidic, Electric, Electronic) control circuits use devices such as valves, nozzles, ducted ejectors, and diaphragms.

23. Fluidic control circuits operate on the principle of the _____ (Fluidic Effect, Halo Effect, Coanda Effect) by using gas flow and pressure to control the ventilator functions.

24. _____ (Electronic, Pneumatic, Fluidic) control circuits use resistors, diodes, transistors, integrated circuits, and sometimes, microprocessors, to control the drive mechanisms of the ventilators.

CONTROL VARIABLES

25. Name the four control variables that may be found on mechanical ventilators.

    _____

    _____

    _____

    _____

26. A ventilator is classified as a pressure controller if the ventilator controls the transrespiratory system _____ (volume, flow, pressure).

27. A positive pressure ventilator applies pressure _____ (inside, outside) the chest to expand the lungs, and it is the type of ventilator most commonly used today.

28. Negative pressure ventilators apply subatmospheric pressure _____ (inside, outside) the chest to inflate the lungs.

29. For ventilators that provide pressure-controlled ventilation, exhalation begins when the _____ (positive, negative, positive or negative) pressure ceases.

30. In mechanical ventilation, exhalation is typically passive and due to the _____ (airflow resistance, elastic recoil) of the lungs.

31. With a pressure controller, the pressure level that is delivered to the patient _____ (will, will not) vary in spite of changes in the patient's compliance or resistance.

32. With a pressure controller, the volume delivered to the patient _____ (will, will not) vary in conditions of changing compliance or resistance. A _____ (larger, smaller) volume results when the compliance is low or the resistance is high.

33. A volume controller allows the _____ (flow, pressure, volume) to vary with changes in resistance and compliance, while keeping the _____ (flow, pressure, volume) delivered constant.

34. With a volume controller, the _____ (flow, pressure, volume) becomes _____ (higher, lower) in conditions of decreasing compliance or increasing resistance.

35. Flow controllers allow _____ (time, flow, pressure) to vary with changes in the patient's compliance and resistance, while directly measuring and controlling the _____ (flow, pressure, volume).

36. With a flow controller, the _____ (flow, pressure, volume) becomes _____ (higher, lower) in conditions of decreasing compliance or increasing resistance.

37. Some mechanical ventilators use _____ (flow and pressure, pressure and inspiratory time, flow and inspiratory time) to generate the tidal volume.

38. Time controllers are ventilators that measure and control the _____ (inspiratory, expiratory, inspiratory and expiratory) time. These ventilators allow _____ (pressure, volume, pressure and volume) to vary with changes in pulmonary compliance and resistance.

PHASE VARIABLES

39. A ventilator breath may be divided into _____ (two, three, four) distinct phases.

40. Describe the phases of a ventilator breath.

_____

_____

_____

41. The trigger variable is a factor that determines the _____ (start, end) of _____ (inspiration, expiration).

42. List three factors that can be used as trigger variables during mechanical ventilation.

_____

_____

_____

43. When a ventilator delivers a breath at a predetermined time interval, the mechanical breath is _____ triggered.

44. When a ventilator uses change in circuit pressure to initiate inspiration, the mechanical breath is _____ triggered.

45. Explain a flow-triggered breath.

_____

_____

46. The amount of work needed to initiate or trigger a ventilator breath is called _____ (peak inspiratory pressure, peak flow, sensitivity).

47. The sensitivity of a ventilator should be set _____ (higher, lower) to make it easier for the patient to trigger a breath. (Note: higher means more sensitive to the patient's needs, lower means less sensitive to the patient's needs.)

48. When one or more (pressure, flow, or volume) variables is not allowed to rise above a preset value during the inspiratory time, it is termed a _____ (trigger, limit, cycle) variable.

49. With a limit variable, inspiration _____ (ends, does not end) when the variable reaches its preset value. The breath delivery _____ (stops, continues) while the variable is held at the fixed, preset value.

50. When the peak pressure reaches a preset value *before* inspiration ends, the breath is _____ (time-, pressure-, flow-, volume-) limited.

51. When the volume reaches a preset value *before* inspiration ends, the breath is _____ (flow-, pressure-, volume-, time-) limited.

52. With a cycle variable, _____ (inspiration, expiration) ends when a specific cycling variable (i.e., pressure, volume, flow, or time) is reached.

53. When the inspiratory flow ends *because* a preset pressure is reached, the breath is _____ (flow-, pressure-, volume-, time-) cycled.

54. When the inspiratory flow ends *because* a preset volume is reached, the breath is _____ (flow-, pressure-, volume-, time-) cycled.

55. A baseline variable is a variable that is controlled during the _____ (inspiratory, expiratory) phase or time.

56. Give two examples of baseline variables.

   _____

   _____

57. Conditional variables are defined as changes detected by the _____ (ventilator, patient) when a certain threshold is met, resulting in a designated _____ (input, output).

TERMINOLOGY OF VENTILATION MODES

58. Volume-controlled ventilation allows the clinician to set the _____ (pressure, volume, pressure and volume). With this mode, the _____ (pressure, volume) will vary depending upon the patient's pulmonary compliance and airway resistance.

59. Pressure-controlled ventilation allows the clinician to set the _____ (pressure, volume, pressure and volume). With this mode, the _____ (pressure, volume) will vary depending upon the patient's pulmonary compliance and airway resistance.

60. Intermittent mandatory ventilation (IMV) _____ (allows, does not allow) the patient to breathe spontaneously between time-triggered ventilator breaths.

61. Pressure support cannot be used when the patient is breathing spontaneously during IMV. _____ (TRUE/FALSE)

62. Pressure support augments a patient's spontaneous tidal volume with a preset _____ (flow, pressure) and a variable _____ (flow, pressure).

63. Dual control within a breath implies that two variables become control variables during the _____ (inspiration phase, expiratory phase, entire respiratory cycle) within the same breath.

64. Dual control breath-to-breath mode allow the clinician to set a _____ (pressure, volume) target, and the ventilator delivers pressure-controlled breaths attempting to achieve the desired target _____ (peak inspiratory pressure, tidal volume).

65. In pressure-limited time-cycled breaths, the clinician sets a target tidal volume and maximum pressure (pressure limit). _____ (TRUE/FALSE)

66. In pressure-limited time-cycled breaths, the _____ (pressure, volume) increases to a set value or target, and inspiration ends _____ (when the pressure limit is reached, at a specified time interval).

67. Pressure-limited flow-cycled breaths start as a _____ (pressure-controlled, pressure-support breath) with a target tidal volume.

68. During pressure-limited flow-cycled breaths, if the tidal volume falls below the target level, the inspiratory pressure is _____ (increased, decreased) on the next breath to attempt to achieve the tidal volume target.

69. With automode, if the patient breathes spontaneously for two consecutive breaths, the ventilator will switch to _____ (volume support ventilation [VSV] mode, pressure-regulated volume control [PRVC] mode). If the patient becomes apneic (12 seconds for adults, 8 seconds for pediatrics), the ventilator will switch back to _____ (volume support ventilation [VSV] mode, pressure-regulated volume control [PRVC] mode).

70. Proportional assist ventilation (PAV) uses an appropriate amount of pressure support that is tailored or adjusted to the patient's spontaneous effort, _____ (increasing, decreasing) the pressure support level when the patient's work of breathing is increased.

71. Automatic tube compensation automatically compensates for the _____ (resistance of the artificial airway, compliance of the lungs). This mode is active during _____ (inspiration, expiration, inspiration and expiration).

72. Airway pressure release ventilation (APRV) is a form of continuous positive airway pressure (CPAP) with _____ (one, two) distinct pressure level(s). It maintains spontaneous breathing throughout the entire ventilatory cycle at _____ (one, both) pressure level(s).

73. During APRV, _____ (oxygenation, removal of CO_2) is enhanced by releasing the pressure from the higher to the lower pressure setting.

74. During APRV, _____ (inspiration, expiration) occurs when the pressure is released from the higher to the lower pressure setting.

OUTPUT WAVEFORMS

75. Name three basic output waveforms during mechanical ventilation.

_____

_____

_____

76. The _____ (rectangular, exponential, sinusoidal, oscillating) pressure waveform is characterized by a near-instantaneous rise to a peak pressure value that is held constant until the start of exhalation, followed by a rapid pressure drop to baseline during exhalation.

77. The _____ (rectangular, exponential, sinusoidal, oscillating) pressure waveform resembles the positive half of a sine wave. These waveforms are produced by ventilators using a _____ (linear-, compressor-, rotary-) driven piston drive mechanism.

78. Name two types of volume waveforms.

_____

_____

79. Name four types of flow waveforms.

_____

_____

_____

_____

ALARM SYSTEMS

80. Input power alarms in mechanical ventilation can be classified as to loss of _____ (electrical, pneumatic power, electrical or pneumatic power).

81. An inappropriate ventilator setting will trigger the _____ (input power, control circuit, output) alarm(s), and this event _____ (allows, does not allow) the clinician to change the input to one that is compatible.

82. What are the five major parameters that output alarms monitor?

_____

_____

_____

_____

_____

83. Airway obstruction is most likely to trigger the _____ (high, low, mean airway, baseline airway) pressure alarm.

84. Circuit disconnection may trigger all of the following pressure alarms *except*:

    A. high pressure alarm.

    B. low pressure alarm.

    C. low volume alarm.

    D. apnea alarm.

85. A _____ (high, low) tidal volume alarm condition may result from oversedation, circuit disconnection, or apnea.

86. Flow alarms are limited to exhaled _____ (peak flow, tidal volume, minute volume).

87. Time alarms are triggered when the inspiratory time or expiratory time is _____ (too long, too short, too long or too short).

88. Inspired gas alarms alert the clinician to changes in gas _____ (concentration, temperature, concentration or temperature).

89. What are the two common gas analyzers used in mechanical ventilation?

    _____

    _____

CHAPTER 4

Operating Modes of Mechanical Ventilation

NEGATIVE AND POSITIVE PRESSURE VENTILATION

1. Most mechanical ventilators deliver flow and volume by creating a _____ pressure gradient between the airway opening and the alveoli.

   A. positive

   B. negative

   C. zero

   D. positive or negative

2. The pressure gradient (difference) between the airway opening and the alveoli is called the:

   A. pleural pressure.

   B. transairway pressure.

   C. transpulmonary pressure.

   D. intrathoracic pressure.

3. Under normal operating conditions, a larger transairway pressure gradient generated by the patient or ventilator creates a _____ (higher, lower) flow or volume.

4. Negative pressure ventilation creates a transairway pressure gradient by _____ (increasing, decreasing) the alveolar pressures to a level _____ (above, below) the airway opening pressure and the atmospheric pressure.

5. Name two negative pressure ventilators.

   _____

   _____

6. An "iron lung" ventilator provides ventilation by creating a negative pressure around the patient's _____ (neck and head, chest cage and abdomen).

7. The tidal volume delivered by a negative pressure ventilator is directly related to the negative pressure gradient. _____ (TRUE/FALSE)

8. Disadvantages and complications of the iron lung ventilator include _____ and _____. (Tank shock is a condition where the venous return to the right atrium is reduced.)

9. Chest cuirass ventilators are often used in a(n) _____ (acute, home) care facility because they are _____ (easy, difficult) to maintain and _____ (can, cannot) be used to provide ventilation without an artificial airway.

10. When a positive pressure ventilator is used, the tidal volume delivered to the patient is directly related to the positive pressure gradient. _____ (TRUE/FALSE)

11. In mechanical ventilation, a larger tidal volume requires a _____ (higher, lower) transairway pressure gradient.

OPERATING MODES OF MECHANICAL VENTILATION

12. _____ describes how the ventilator adjusts its output to suit a patient's changing variable.

13. In pressure support, the input (pressure set by the clinician) is constant and the output (flow delivered by the ventilator) is variable, depending on the changing characteristics of the airways and lungs. Pressure support is considered a(n) _____ (open-loop, closed-loop) system.

14. In the spontaneous mode, the work of breathing is provided by the _____ (ventilator, patient).

15. Positive end-expiratory pressure (PEEP) increases the end-expiratory or baseline airway pressure to a value greater than _____ (−3, 0, 3) cm H_2O. It is used to manage _____ (hypercapnia, hypoxemia, refractory hypoxemia) caused by _____ (hypoventilation, V/Q mismatch, intrapulmonary shunting).

16. When PEEP is applied to spontaneously breathing patients (without mechanical breaths), the airway pressure is called _____.

17. Three indications for PEEP are _____ (V/Q mismatch, intrapulmonary shunting), _____ (increased, decreased) functional residual capacity and _____ (auto-PEEP, CPAP) compensation.

18. In the presence of auto-PEEP that does not respond to adjustments of ventilator settings, PEEP may be set slightly _____ (above, below) the auto-PEEP level. This raises the end-expiratory baseline pressure and reduces the _____ (spontaneous frequency, breath-triggering effort).

19. Refractory hypoxemia is likely to be present when the PaO_2 is _____ mm Hg or less at an F_IO_2 of _____ % or higher.

20. PEEP provides positive pressure to the lung parenchyma at the _____ (beginning, end) of _____ (inhalation, exhalation) until the next respiratory cycle. It _____ (increases, decreases) the functional residual capacity, _____ (increases, lowers) the required alveolar distending pressure, and improves oxygenation.

21. A patient has been using PEEP at levels between 15 and 18 cm H_2O. The physician asks the therapist to monitor the potential adverse effects caused by PEEP. The therapist should monitor all of the following conditions *except*:

    A. decreased venous return.

    B. increased cardiac output and renal perfusion.

    C. barotrauma.

    D. increased intracranial pressure.

22. Venous return to the _____ (left, right) atrium is influenced by the pressure gradient between the central venous pressure and the negative pleural pressure that surrounds the heart. During PEEP, the pleural pressure becomes _____ (more, less) negative and the pressure gradient will decrease, resulting in a(n) _____ (increased, decreased) venous return and cardiac output.

23. The effects of PEEP on the venous return are the same regardless of the compliance characteristic of the patient. _____ (TRUE/FALSE)

24. The adverse effects of PEEP on the venous return and cardiac output are _____ (more, less) severe on patients with low lung compliance than those with normal compliance.

25. The incidence of barotrauma is increased when PEEP is higher than _____ (10, 15, 20) cm H_2O, mean airway pressure is higher than _____ (20, 30, 40) cm H_2O, and peak inspiratory pressure is higher than _____ (40, 50, 60) cm H_2O.

26. In patients with normal lung compliance, PEEP may _____ (increase, decrease) the intracranial pressure due to impedance of _____ (arterial flow to, venous return from) the head (superior vena cava).

27. Positive pressure ventilation can _____ (increase, reduce) the blood flow to the kidneys. As a result, the urine output is _____ (increased, decreased) as the kidneys try to correct the perceived _____ (hypervolemic, hypovolemic) condition by _____ (retaining, secreting) fluid.

CONTINUOUS POSITIVE AIRWAY PRESSURE

28. Continuous positive airway pressure (CPAP) is _____ (PEEP, oxygen, air) applied to the airway of a patient who is breathing spontaneously.

29. The indications for CPAP are essentially the same as for PEEP, with the additional requirement that the patient must have adequate spontaneous ventilation documented by the _____ (pH, $PaCO_2$, PaO_2) measurements.

BI-LEVEL POSITIVE AIRWAY PRESSURE

30. Bi-level positive airway pressure (BiPAP) may be used to prevent intubation of the patients with end-stage COPD and to support patients with chronic ventilatory failure. _____ (TRUE/FALSE)

31. In patients who are breathing spontaneously, the initial IPAP and EPAP may be set at _____ (4, 6, 8) cm H_2O and _____ (4, 6, 8) cm H_2O, respectively, and the backup rate may be set at 2 to 5 breaths _____ (above, below) the patient's spontaneous rate.

32. When BiPAP is used in the timed (control) mode, the rate is usually set slightly _____ (higher, lower) than the patient's spontaneous rate.

33. A BiPAP device can be used as a CPAP device by setting the IPAP and EPAP at the same level. _____ (TRUE/FALSE)

34. In general, the IPAP is adjusted in 2-cm H_2O increments to regulate the patient's _____ (oxygenation, acid-base balance, ventilation), and the EPAP is adjusted in 2-cm H_2O increments to regulate the patient's _____ (oxygenation, acid-base balance, alveolar ventilation).

CONTROLLED MANDATORY VENTILATION (CMV)

35. With controlled mandatory ventilation, a patient _____ (can, cannot) increase the ventilator frequency or breath spontaneously.

36. The control mode may be used any time without the use of sedatives, respiratory depressants, and neuromuscular blockers. _____ (TRUE/FALSE)

37. The _____ (spontaneous, control) mode is more likely to develop rapid disuse atrophy of the diaphragm fibers.

ASSIST/CONTROL

38. With an assist/control (AC) mode, each control breath provides a _____ (spontaneous, mechanical) tidal volume, and each assist breath results in a _____ (spontaneous, mechanical) tidal volume.

39. While on the AC mode, the patient has a stable and regular assist frequency of 16/min, the ventilator has a control rate of 12/min, and the total frequency is _____ (12, 16, 28) breaths per minute.

40. The AC mode is typically used for patients who have a(n) _____ (stable, unstable) respiratory drive and _____ (can, cannot) trigger the ventilator into inspiration. Therefore, the ventilator frequency is usually set at 2 to 4 breaths per minute _____ (above, below) the patient's assist frequency.

41. The AC mode _____ (allows, does not allow) the patient to control the frequency and therefore the minute volume required to normalize the $PaCO_2$.

42. The potential hazard associated with the AC mode is alveolar hypoventilation and respiratory acidosis. _____ (TRUE/FALSE)

INTERMITTENT MANDATORY VENTILATION

43. Intermittent mandatory ventilation (IMV) is a mode in which the ventilator delivers _____ (assist, control) breaths and allows the patient to breathe spontaneously at _____ (a preset, any) tidal volume in between the mandatory breaths.

44. In the IMV mode, if the mandatory breaths are delivered at a frequency independent of the patient's spontaneous frequency, breath stacking may be a problem. _____ (TRUE/FALSE)

SYNCHRONIZED INTERMITTENT MANDATORY VENTILATION (SIMV)

45. Synchronized intermittent mandatory ventilation (SIMV) is a mode in which the ventilator delivers control (mandatory) breaths to the patient at or near the _____ (beginning, end) of a spontaneous breath.

46. The SIMV mandatory breaths may be either time-triggered or patient-triggered, and these mandatory breaths are delivered to the patient at _____ (regular, variable) intervals.

47. When a patient is breathing spontaneously at a SIMV frequency of 12/min, a mandatory breath occurs _____ (at precisely, at or about) every _____ (2, 3, 5, 6, 10) sec.

48. SIMV is a mode in which the ventilator delivers _____ (assist, control) breaths and allows the patient to breathe spontaneously at _____ (a preset, any) tidal volume in between the mandatory breaths.

49. Since SIMV promotes spontaneous breathing and use of respiratory muscles, all of the following are potential advantages of the SIMV mode *except*:

    A. decreased work of breathing.

    B. preventing atrophy of respiratory muscles.

    C. decreased mean airway pressure.

    D. reduced V/Q mismatch.

MANDATORY MINUTE VENTILATION (MVV)

50. Mandatory minute ventilation (MMV), also called minimum minute ventilation, is a feature on some ventilators that provides a predetermined _____ (peak inspiratory pressure, pressure support level, minute ventilation) when the patient's spontaneous breathing effort becomes _____ (excessive, inadequate).

51. MMV is a feature on some ventilators that helps to prevent _____ (hypocapnia, hypercapnia) due to _____ (excessive, inadequate) spontaneous ventilation.

52. A minute volume maintained by rapid spontaneous frequency and low tidal volume (e.g., distressed patient) may avert the MMV function but at the same time will result in a significant amount of deadspace ventilation. _____ (TRUE/FALSE)

53. During MMV, a minute volume maintained by rapid spontaneous frequency and low tidal volume may _____ (trigger, avert) the MMV function. This breathing pattern increases the amount of _____ (deadspace ventilation, spontaneous tidal volume).

PRESSURE SUPPORT VENTILATION (PSV)

54. Pressure support ventilation (PSV) is used to increase the work of spontaneous breathing. _____ (TRUE/FALSE)

55. PSV is commonly used during the weaning process because PSV _____ (increases, decreases) the patient's work of breathing.

56. When PSV is working as intended, it _____ (increases, decreases) the patient's spontaneous tidal volume and _____ (increases, decreases) the spontaneous frequency.

57. The initial pressure support level may be titrated until the spontaneous tidal volume equals _____ mL/kg or the spontaneous frequency is less than _____/min.

58. When a pressure support breath is triggered, the ventilator rapidly increases the airway pressure to _____ (10 cm H_2O, 30 cm H_2O, the preset pressure support level).

59. In PSV, the inspiratory pressure plateau is maintained at the same level until the:

    A. spontaneous tidal volume is more than 400 mL.

    B. end-flow drops to a predetermined level (e.g., 5 L/min).

    C. pressure support level is less than 10 cm H_2O.

    D. all of the above.

ADAPTIVE SUPPORT VENTILATION

60. In adaptive support ventilation (ASV) mode, the therapist needs to input the patient's _____ (arterial blood gas results, body weight, height) and the desired _____ (percent minute ventilation, $PaCO_2$, peak inspiratory pressure).

61. When ASV mode is used on adults, the ventilator uses a predetermined minute ventilation setting of _____ (20, 50, 100, 200) mL/min/kg.

62. If the therapist inputs a body weight of 50 kg and 150% as the desired minute ventilation for an adult patient, the resulting minute ventilation would be _____ (2,500, 5,000, 7,500) mL.

63. When ASV mode is used on children, the ventilator uses a predetermined minute ventilation setting of _____ (20, 50, 100, 200) mL/min/kg.

64. If the therapist inputs a body weight of 20 kg and 100% as the desired minute ventilation for a child, the resulting minute ventilation would be _____ (200, 400, 2,000, 4,000) mL.

65. With ASV, the ventilator changes the _____ according to the patient's breathing pattern.

    A. number of mandatory breaths

    B. pressure support level

    C. percent minute ventilation

    D. A and B only

66. If there is no spontaneous breathing effort during ASV, the ventilator would determine and provide the:

    A. mandatory frequency.

    B. tidal volume.

    C. I:E ratio.

    D. all of the above.

67. When the patient increases the triggering effort during ASV, the number of _____ (spontaneous, mandatory) breaths decreases and the _____ (ventilator frequency, ventilator tidal volume, pressure support) increases.

PROPORTIONAL ASSIST VENTILATION (PAV)

68. Proportional assist ventilation (PAV) is a mode of ventilation that changes the _____ (pressure support, tidal volume, peak inspiratory pressure) level according to the patient's volume, elastance, airflow resistance, and flow demand.

69. PAV is active in a(n) _____ (assist, mandatory) breath only, and the breath may provide _____ (flow assist, volume assist, flow or volume assist).

70. In volume support (VS), PAV provides the pressure to meet the patient's _____ (pressure, flow, volume) requirement.

71. The pressure provided by PAV may be too _____ (high, low) in conditions where the elastance and airflow resistance shows sudden *improvement*. This change may lead to _____ (overdistention, atelectasis).

VOLUME-ASSURED PRESSURE SUPPORT (VAPS)

72. Volume-assured pressure support (VAPS) is a mode of ventilation that assures a stable _____ (peak inspiratory pressure, tidal volume) by combining pressure support and _____ (pressure-assisted cycles, volume-assisted cycles).

73. In VAPS, the therapist needs to preset the _____ (minimal tidal volume, pressure support, minimal tidal volume and pressure support) level.

74. During VAPS, the mechanical breaths are _____ (patient-, time-, patient- or time-) triggered.

75. In VAPS, the volume delivered by pressure support should be titrated to a point that is _____ (higher than, same as, lower than) the preset minimal tidal volume.

76. If the delivered volume during VAPS falls short of the preset tidal volume, the ventilator switches from a _____ (pressure-limited, volume-limited) breath to a _____ (pressure-limited, volume-limited) breath.

77. If the delivered volume during VAPS falls short of the preset tidal volume, the ventilator uses a _____ (longer, shorter) inspiratory time at a _____ (variable, constant) flow until the preset volume is delivered.

78. Since VAPS may prolong the inspiratory time, patients with _____ (restrictive lung disorder, airflow obstruction) should be monitored closely in order to prevent air trapping and other related side effects.

PRESSURE-REGULATED VOLUME CONTROL (PRVC)

79. Pressure-regulated volume control (PRVC) on the _____ (Servo 300®, Hamilton Galileo®, Evita 4®) ventilator is active in the CMV mode only.

80. PRVC provides volume support (VS) with the lowest pressure possible by changing the _____ (pressure support, flow and inspiratory time, tidal volume).

81. When increase in airflow resistance is encountered during PRVC, the ventilator uses a lower inspiratory flow to reduce the _____ (peak inspiratory, plateau, mean airway) pressure.

82. When increase in airflow resistance is encountered during PRVC, a lower flow requires a compensatory _____ (longer, shorter) inspiratory time to deliver the preset tidal volume.

83. In automode, the Servo 300A ventilator provides a _____ (flow-triggered, pressure-triggered, time-triggered) breath when prolonged apnea is detected.

ADAPTIVE PRESSURE CONTROL (APC)

84. Adaptive pressure control (APC) offers a dual-control mechanism that combines the functions of volume ventilation (via stable _____ [frequency, tidal volume]) with the functions of pressure ventilation (via _____ [stable, variable] flow).

85. With APC, as the patient's inspiratory effort increases, the inflation pressure is _____ (increased, reduced). This is a concern because the ventilator _____ (can, cannot) distinguish between improved pulmonary compliance and increased patient effort.

VOLUME VENTILATION PLUS (VV+)

86. What are the two dual mode volume-targeted breath types in volume ventilation plus (VV+) on a Puritan Bennett 840® ventilator?

_____

_____

87. In volume control plus (VC+), the therapist sets the _____ (target tidal volume, inspiratory time, target tidal volume and inspiratory time).

88. In VC+ the target pressures following the test breath are adjusted accordingly to compensate for any _____ (tidal volume, airway pressure) differences.

89. In VC+, the inspiratory flow is _____ (constant, variable).

90. During the inspiratory phase of a VC+ mandatory breath, spontaneous breaths _____ (are, are not) allowed.

91. In VS, the therapist sets the _____ (target tidal volume, inspiratory time, mandatory rate).

92. In VS, the ventilator uses variable _____ (flow, peak inspiratory pressure, pressure support) levels to provide the target tidal volume.

93. As the patient assumes a higher spontaneous tidal volume during VS, the ventilator _____ (increases, decreases) the pressure support level accordingly.

PRESSURE CONTROL VENTILATION (PCV)

94. In pressure control ventilation (PCV), the pressure-controlled breaths are typically _____ (patient-, time-) triggered, and therefore the frequency is _____ (variable, preset).

95. PCV is usually indicated for patients with severe ARDS who require extremely high _____ (PEEP, peak inspiratory pressure) during volume-controlled ventilation.

96. The advantage of switching these patients from the conventional volume-controlled ventilation to pressure-controlled ventilation is that a _____ (higher, lower) peak inspiratory pressure can be attained while maintaining sufficient oxygenation (PaO_2) and ventilation ($PaCO_2$).

97. Since PCV is controlled by the preset pressure limit, the tidal volume delivered to the patient will decrease with _____ (increasing, decreasing) lung compliance or _____ (increasing, decreasing) airway resistance.

AIRWAY PRESSURE RELEASE VENTILATION (APRV)

98. Airway pressure release ventilation (APRV) has _____ (one, two, three) CPAP or pressure level(s).

99. APRV has a high pressure (P_{high} or P_{INSP}) and a low pressure (P_{low} or PEEP), and the patient is allowed to breathe spontaneously _____ (with some, without) restriction.

100. In APRV, when the high pressure (P_{high}) level is dropped or "released" to the low pressure (P_{low}) level, it simulates a mechanical _____ (inspiration, expiration). When the low pressure (P_{low}) level is raised to the high pressure (P_{high}) level, it simulates an _____ (inspiratory, expiratory) mechanical breath.

101. In APRV, the patient spends most of the time at the _____ (high, low) pressure level with less than 1.5 sec at the _____ (high, low) pressure level.

102. During APRV, the patient is allowed to breathe spontaneously at the _____ (high pressure level only, low pressure level only, high or low pressure levels).

103. The primary indication for APRV is similar to that of pressure-controlled ventilation—limiting the high peak inspiratory pressure while under volume-controlled ventilation. _____ (TRUE/FALSE)

BIPHASIC POSITIVE AIRWAY PRESSURE (BIPHASIC PAP)

104. Biphasic PAP is similar to APRV, with one exception. In APRV, the patient spends most of the time at the _____ (high, low) pressure level with less than 1.5 sec at the low pressure level. In biphasic PAP, the patient spends more time at the _____ (high, low) pressure level.

INVERSE RATIO VENTILATION (IRV)

105. Inverse ratio ventilation (IRV) improves oxygenation by all of the following mechanisms *except*:

     A. reduction of intrapulmonary shunting.

     B. improvement of V/Q matching.

     C. increase of deadspace ventilation.

     D. enhancement of alveolar recruitment.

106. With a longer inspiratory time than expiratory time, IRV tends to cause a _____ (higher, lower) mean airway pressure and development of _____ (atelectasis, intrapulmonary shunting, auto-PEEP).

107. The increase in mean airway pressure and development of auto-PEEP during IRV help to reduce shunting and improve oxygenation in ARDS patients. _____ (TRUE/FALSE)

108. During IRV, the increase in mPaw leads to a higher incidence of _____ (intrapulmonary shunting, deadspace ventilation, barotrauma).

109. Sedation and neuromuscular blocking agents are often needed to facilitate ventilation in patients receiving IRV. _____ (TRUE/FALSE)

110. Since IRV tends to _____ (increase, decrease) the mean airway pressure, create auto-PEEP, and increase the incidence of barotrauma, it is sometimes used with pressure control to reduce the airway pressures.

111. When _____ (pressure control, pressure support) is used with IRV, it is called pressure control inverse ratio ventilation (PC-IRV).

AUTOMATIC TUBE COMPENSATION (ATC)

112. Automatic tube compensation (ATC) offsets and compensates for the _____ (lung compliance, airflow resistance, lung compliance and airflow resistance) imposed by the artificial airway.

113. ATC allows the patient to have a breathing pattern as if breathing spontaneously without an artificial airway. _____ (TRUE/FALSE)

NEURALLY ADJUSTED VENTILATORY ASSIST (NAVA)

114. Neurally adjusted ventilatory assist (NAVA) is a mode of mechanical ventilation in which the patient's electrical activity of the _____ (brain, lungs, diaphragm) is used to guide the optimal functions of the ventilator.

115. NAVA is available for adults only. _____ (TRUE/FALSE)

HIGH-FREQUENCY OSCILLATORY VENTILATION (HFOV)

116. In high-frequency oscillatory ventilation (HFOV), ventilation can be increased by _____ (increasing, decreasing) the oscillation frequency.

117. In addition to *decreasing* the oscillation frequency of HFOV, ventilation can also be increased by _____ (increasing, decreasing) the amplitude of the oscillations, inspiratory time, or bias flow (with an intentional cuff leak).

118. In HFOV, oxygenation to the patient can be increased by increasing the F_IO_2 or the _____ (peak inspiratory pressure, mean airway pressure, PEEP).

CHAPTER 5

Special Airways
for Ventilation

INTRODUCTION

1. The oropharyngeal airway, nasopharyngeal airway, esophageal obturator airway (EOA), esophageal gastric tube airway (EGTA), laryngeal mask airway (LMA), esophageal-tracheal Combitube (ETC), and double-lumen endotracheal tube (DLT) are special airways for the purpose of facilitating _____ (drug administration, ventilation, ventilation and oxygenation).

OROPHARYNGEAL AIRWAY

2. An oropharyngeal airway may be used to relieve upper airway obstruction or as a bite block in intubated patients. _____ (TRUE/FALSE)

3. An oropharyngeal airway should not be used in patients who are _____ (conscious, unconscious, sedated) because this airway may stimulate the gag reflex and cause vomiting and aspiration.

4. An oropharyngeal airway may induce gag reflex, vomiting, and aspiration when it is used in _____ (conscious, unconscious) patients.

5. The Berman airways _____ (have, do not have) side channels, and they range from size _____ (43 mm, 60 mm, 80 mm) for infants to size _____ (110 mm, 140 mm, 160 mm) for extra-large adults.

6. The Guedel airway (regular or Cath-Guide) may have _____ (one, three, one or three) _____ [side channel(s), internal channel(s)].

7. Guedel airways have sizes ranging from _____ (24 mm, 55 mm, 76 mm) for infants to _____ (100 mm, 120 mm, 160 mm) for extra-large adults.

8. The appropriate size (from flange to distal tip) of an oropharyngeal airway may be estimated based on the length in mm from the _____ (corner, center) of the mouth to the angle of the jaw.

9. Another way to estimate the appropriate size of an oropharyngeal airway is to measure the length in mm from the corner of the mouth to the _____ (angle of the jaw, earlobe).

10. The third method to estimate the appropriate size of an oropharyngeal airway is to measure the distance from the central incisors to the _____ (earlobe, angle of the jaw, top of the forehead).

11. If the patient begins to gag or retch during insertion of an oropharyngeal airway, the airway should be _____ (turned upside down to facilitate insertion, removed immediately because the patient might not need an airway).

12. A properly inserted oropharyngeal airway should have the flange resting _____ (on the patient's lips or teeth, completely inside the patient's mouth).

NASOPHARYNGEAL AIRWAY

13. A nasopharyngeal airway _____ (can, cannot) be used in patients with an intact gag reflex.

14. Indications for a nasopharyngeal airway include all of the following *except*:

    A. fractures of the mandible.

    B. trimus (lockjaw).

    C. nasal trauma.

    D. oral trauma.

15. The appropriate size of nasopharyngeal airway for average females is a size _____ (4, 6, 8), and average males a size _____ (5, 7, 9).

16. _____ (Water, Water-soluble lubricant, Petroleum jelly) should be used to facilitate insertion of the nasopharyngeal airway.

ESOPHAGEAL OBTURATOR AIRWAY

17. An EOA is inserted into the _____ (trachea, esophagus), and it is a _____ (reusable, disposable) tube.

18. The EOA has an opening at the _____ (proximal or top, distal or bottom) end, many small holes near the upper end of the tube, and a(n) _____ (open, closed) distal end.

19. Near the distal end of an EOA is a _____ (large, small) cuff, which is kept _____ (inflated, deflated) during use.

20. The _____ (inflated, deflated) cuff of an EOA prevents air from entering the stomach, and subsequent regurgitation and aspiration.

21. A mask is used in conjunction with the EOA to:

    A. prevent gas leak around the patient's face during ventilation.

    B. increase oxygen delivery.

    C. provide positive end-expiratory pressure during ventilation.

    D. provide larger tidal volume during ventilation.

22. The small holes at the hypopharyngeal level of an EOA:

    A. prevent regurgitation and aspiration.

    B. provide ventilation to the lungs.

    C. increase the oxygen level.

    D. reduce the deadspace volume.

23. Since an EOA is inserted into the _____ (trachea, esophagus), the cuff at the distal end of the tube must be _____ (inflated, deflated) at all times.

24. Prior to insertion, the cuff of an EOA is inflated with _____ (5 to 10, 10 to 20, 20 to 30, 30 to 40) mL of air to check for cuff integrity and leaks.

25. Arrange the following four steps in the proper order of preparing an EOA tube for use. _____ (D, A, B, C) or (B, A, C, D) or (B, D, A, C)

    A. Lubricate tube with a water-soluble lubricant

    B. Inflate and test cuff

    C. Insert tube through opening of a mask

    D. Deflate cuff

26. Asphyxia and tracheal damage are severe complications if the cuff of an EOA is _____ (inflated, deflated) while the tube is misplaced in the trachea.

27. An EOA:

    A. should be used in awake or semiconscious patients.

    B. should not be used in children under 16 years old or under 5 ft tall.

    C. may be used in patients with known esophageal disease.

    D. may be removed before patient regains consciousness.

28. The EOA _____ (is, is not) designed to be used as an artificial airway for positive pressure ventilation.

29. If the EOA is to be replaced with an endotracheal tube, endotracheal intubation should be performed _____ (after removal of EOA, with EOA in place).

ESOPHAGEAL GASTRIC TUBE AIRWAY

30. The major difference between an EOA and an EGTA is that an EOA has a(n) _____ (open, closed) distal end and an EGTA has a(n) _____ (open, closed) distal end.

31. The advantage of an EGTA is its capability of relieving gastric distention that may occur during bag-to-mask ventilation. _____ (TRUE/FALSE)

32. With an EGTA, ventilation holes along the proximal end of the tube are _____ (absent, present), and ventilation is provided through the _____ (adapter, mask) by a traditional manual resuscitation bag.

33. Since there are two ports on the ETGA mask, the resuscitation bag must be attached to the _____ (gastric, ventilation) port.

34. Distinct features of EOA and EGTA include: EOA and EGTA are both inserted into the _____ (esophagus, trachea); only _____ (EOA, EGTA) has ventilation holes along its tube; only _____ (EOA, EGTA) has a patent distal end; only _____ (EOA, EGTA) has two ports on the mask.

LARYNGEAL MASK AIRWAY

35. The LMA resembles a _____ (long, short) endotracheal tube with a small, cushioned, oblong-shaped _____ (cuff, mask) on the distal end.

36. A properly inserted LMA provides a seal over the _____ (vocal cords, esophagus, trachea, laryngeal opening), and it _____ (is, is not) necessary for the LMA to enter the larynx or trachea.

37. The LMA can withstand positive pressures of up to _____ (10, 20, 30, 40) cm H_2O. (Note: up to 30 cm H_2O with LMA-Proseal.)

38. The LMA is suitable to use during resuscitation in the _____ (conscious, unconscious) patient with _____ (active, absent) glossopharyngeal and laryngeal reflexes.

39. Complete the following statements on the uses of an LMA: LMA intubation _____ (is, is not) a suitable option following failed endotracheal intubation attempts; LMA _____ (may, may not) be used in infants and children; LMA provides _____ (higher, lower) airflow resistance and work of breathing than an endotracheal tube.

40. The LMA _____ (is, is not) capable of protecting an airway from the effects of regurgitation and aspiration.

41. Since the LMA can withhold pressures only up to _____ (10, 20, 30) cm H_2O, a leak may occur during high airway pressure situations. Patients with _____ (high, low) airway resistance or _____ (high, low) lung compliance should use an endotracheal tube.

42. The reusable LMA is made with _____ (silicone, polyvinyl chloride).

43. For most adults, a size _____ (3, 4, 5, 6) LMA should be used for females and size _____ (3, 4, 5, 6) for males.

44. The standard cuff pressure for an LMA is _____ (30, 40, 50, 60) cm H_2O, and it is adjusted accordingly to decrease the intracuff pressure.

45 to 52. Write in the recommended size of an LMA for each respective patient group.

SIZE	PATIENT GROUP
45. _____	Neonates and infants up to 5 kg
46. _____	Infants between 5 and 10 kg
47. _____	Infants and children between 10 and 20 kg

48. _____   Children between 20 and 30 kg

49. _____   Children over 30 kg and small adults

50. _____   Adults 50 to 70 kg

51. _____   Adults 70 to 100 kg

52. _____   Adults over 100 kg

53. The LMA is inserted _____ (with, without) a laryngoscope through the mouth and advanced along the hard palate. It is then further advanced to the _____ (posterior pharynx, vocal cords) and turned toward the _____ (pharynx, esophagus, trachea and larynx).

54. The LMA may be removed when the patient is _____ (anesthetized, awake, anesthetized or awake).

55. List at least three complications that may occur during removal of an LMA.

   _____

   _____

   _____

56. Rotation or turning of the LMA may cause misplacement of the mask and result in gastric insufflation and air leakage from the mask seal. _____ (TRUE/FALSE)

57. Reusable LMAs are sterilized by _____ (liquid sterilizing agent, steam autoclave, radiation).

ESOPHAGEAL-TRACHEAL COMBITUBE (ETC)

58. An ETC is a combination of _____ and _____ in one unit.

59. The ETC is inserted into the _____ (esophagus, trachea, esophagus or trachea).

60. There _____ (is one, are two) cuff(s) on the ETC.

61. On the ETC, a proximal latex pharyngeal cuff holds _____ (15, 100) mL of air, and a PVC cuff near the distal end of the tube holds _____ (15, 100) mL of air.

62. Lumen 1 is used to provide ventilation when the ETC tube enters the _____ (esophagus, trachea), and the _____ (proximal, distal) cuff seals off the _____ (esophagus, trachea).

63. Lumen 2 is used to provide ventilation when the ETC tube enters the _____ (esophagus, trachea), and the _____ (proximal, distal) cuff seals off the _____ (esophagus, trachea).

64. An ETC is inserted _____ (with, without, with or without) a laryngoscope.

65. The ETC is properly inserted once the black rings on the tube lie opposite the _____.

66. After insertion of the ETC, the _____ (distal, proximal, distal and proximal) cuff(s) is (are) inflated immediately.

67. Since ETC is more likely to enter the _____ (esophagus, trachea) during blind intubation, ventilation through the ETC should be done via lumen _____ (1, 2) first.

68. When the distal end of ETC is in the _____ (esophagus, trachea), air goes through the side ports, becomes trapped between the cuffs, and is forced into the trachea.

69. If ventilation via lumen 1 is poor, lumen 2 should be used to provide ventilation, as the distal end of ETC may be in the _____ (esophagus, trachea).

70. If ventilation is poor with lumens 1 and 2, a cuff leak may be present, and this problem may be corrected by inflating the _____ (distal, proximal) cuff with more air.

71. Complications with an ETC are related to either hemodynamic stress or air leaks. _____ (TRUE/FALSE)

DOUBLE-LUMEN ENDOTRACHEAL TUBE (DLT)

72. A double-lumen endobronchial tube (DLT) has _____ (one tracheal and one bronchial, two bronchial) lumens, _____ (one, two) cuff(s), and _____ (one, two) pilot balloon(s).

73. A double-lumen endobronchial is a _____ (left-sided, right-sided, left- or right-sided) tube.

74. The _____ (left-sided, right-sided) DLT is more commonly used because precise placement of the _____ (left-sided, right-sided) tube is more difficult, because the respective upper lobe bronchus is only about 2 cm from the carina of an adult.

75. During insertion, it is more likely for the _____ (left-sided, right-sided) DLT to go past the respective upper lobe bronchus.

76. Which of the following is not an application of independent lung ventilation provided via a DLT?

    A. Reduction of deadspace ventilation

    B. Isolation of left or right lung

    C. Facilitation of lung surgery

    D. Ventilation in bronchopleural or bronchocutaneous fistula

77. If the bronchi are not visible on the chest radiography, the diameter of the left bronchus may be estimated by using _____ (50%, 68%, 75%, 90%) of the tracheal diameter.

78. Adult left-sided DLTs range from _____ (28 to 32 Fr, 35 to 41 Fr, 45 to 50 Fr).

79. The DLT is inserted into the trachea using _____ (blind intubation technique, direct laryngoscopy) _____ (with, without, with or without) a bronchial stylet.

80. When the tracheal cuff of a DLT is just below the vocal cords, the DLT is about _____ (3 cm, 6 cm, 10 cm) from the final position.

81. If a stylet is used to guide the insertion of a DLT, it should be removed _____ (before, as soon as) the DLT has passed the vocal cords, in order to _____ (facilitate successful intubation, minimize the incidence of airway trauma).

82. During insertion of a DLT, the bronchial cuff may be inflated while it is in the trachea to ventilate _____ (the left lung, the right lung, both lungs).

83. When the bronchial tube enters the main-stem bronchus, all of the following may be noticeable *except*:

    A. resistance to advancement.

    B. increase in expired tidal volume.

    C. unilateral ventilation by observation and auscultation.

    D. increase in peak inspiratory pressure (PIP) with volume-controlled ventilation.

84. Once the bronchial plugging point has been identified, the bronchial cuff is _____ (inflated, deflated) and the tube _____ (withdrawn, advanced) another 2.5 to 3 cm.

85. The final bronchial cuff volume is typically about _____ (1 to 2 mL, 3 to 4 mL, 6 to 8 mL).

86. The tracheal cuff is _____ (inflated, deflated) following correct placement of the bronchial cuff.

87. The incidence of airway rupture is higher when large and medium _____ (PVC, red rubber) or _____ small (PVC, red rubber) DLTs are used.

88. Some recommendations for the safe placement of a DLT include:

    A. Choose the _____ (largest, smallest) PVC DLT that is appropriate for the patient.

    B. _____ (Keep, Remove) the bronchial stylet once the tip of the tube is past the vocal cords.

    C. _____ (Always, Never) overinflate both cuffs and use a _____ (3-mL, 10-mL) syringe to inflate the bronchial cuff.

    D. When nitrous oxide is used, measure the cuff pressures intermittently, and keep the bronchial pressure _____ (<30 cm H_2O, >40 cm H_2O).

    E. Deflate the _____ (tracheal cuff, bronchial cuff) when lung isolation is not required.

CHAPTER 6

Airway Management in Mechanical Ventilation

INTUBATION

1. Endotracheal (ET) intubation is done by placing an ET tube inside the trachea through the _____ (mouth, nostril, mouth or nostril).

2. _____ (Tracheostomy, Tracheotomy) is a surgical procedure that creates an airway opening by cutting into the trachea, whereas _____ (tracheostomy, tracheotomy) is the opening thus created.

3. Compared to an ET tube, a tracheostomy tube is _____ (shorter, longer) and provides closer access to the lower airways.

4. In most emergency situations, _____ (ET intubation, tracheotomy) is the preferred procedure to establish an artificial airway.

5. The decision to perform ET intubation versus tracheotomy is based on the patient's _____ (admitting diagnosis, expected duration of needs, age, and weight).

6. Mr. Lang is admitted to the intensive care unit for severe head and chest injuries. He is expected to require mechanical ventilation for the duration, and his recovery time is expected to be lengthy. Based on this information, a(n) _____ (endotracheal, tracheostomy) tube is indicated.

7. The indications for ET intubation include all of the following *except*:

   A. prevention of aspiration.

   B. alleviation of airway obstruction.

   C. removal of secretions.

   D. correction of respiratory alkalosis.

8 to 11. Match the indications for artificial airway with the respective examples. Use each answer only *once*.

INDICATION	EXAMPLE
8. _____ Relief of airway obstruction	A. Loss of swallow or gag reflex
9. _____ Protection of the airway	B. Excessive secretions
10. _____ Facilitation of suctioning	C. Epiglottitis
11. _____ Support of ventilation	D. Mechanical ventilation

COMMON ARTIFICIAL AIRWAYS IN MECHANICAL VENTILATION

12. _____ (Oral intubation, Nasal intubation, Tracheotomy) is easy to perform, and it is the artificial airway of choice in emergency situations.

13. The _____ (largest, smallest) ET tube that is appropriate to the patient's size should be used because it offers _____ (more, less) airflow resistance and imposes _____ (more, less) work of breathing on the patient.

14. In comparison to nasal intubation, oral intubation:

    A. is less likely to cause gagging.

    B. produces less secretion.

    C. is better tolerated by the patient.

    D. allows passage of a larger ET tube.

15. Which of the following is *not* associated with nasal intubation?

    A. Use of a smaller ET tube

    B. Easier to insert than oral intubation

    C. Potential of sinusitis

    D. Use of Magill forceps

16. A tracheostomy tube allows the patient to eat and drink with the tracheostomy cuff properly _____ (inflated, deflated).

17. Infection is most likely to occur in patients whose artificial airway is provided by a(n) _____ (nasal ET tube, oral ET tube, tracheostomy tube). _____ (Good hand-washing, Aseptic, Sterile) techniques must be followed to minimize the incidence of infection.

18. A foam cuff is _____ (inflated by a syringe, self-inflating). Deflation of a foam cuff requires use of a syringe.

19. The tracheostomy button is used to maintain the stoma of a patient on a _____ (temporary, permanent, temporary or permanent) basis.

INTUBATION PROCEDURE

20. Potential contraindications for ET intubation include all of the following conditions *except*:

    A. cervical spine injury.

    B. chest trauma.

    C. airway burns.

    D. facial trauma.

21. Mallampati classification is done by bronchoscopic inspection of the wide-open mouth with the tongue protruded. _____ (TRUE/FALSE)

22. Mallampati classification ranges from class _____ (1 to 3, 1 to 4) where class _____ (1, 3, 4) predicts the maximum difficulty during oral intubation.

23. In Mallampati class 3, the _____ are visible.

    A. soft palate and base of uvula

    B. anterior and posterior tonsillar pillars

    C. fauces and uvula

    D. A and B only

24. Emergency or elective intubation may be done without anesthesia consult in Mallampati class _____ (1 or 2, 2 or 3, 3 or 4).

25. Among the four devices listed below, which is considered optional (least essential) for intubating and managing an oral ET tube?

    A. Laryngoscope handle and blade

    B. 10-mL syringe

    C. Tape

    D. Stylet

26. The laryngoscope handle is typically held by the _____ (left, right) hand.

27. A laryngoscope blade comes in a _____ (straight, curved, straight or curved) design, and these blades range in size from _____ to _____.

28. The Miller blade is a _____ (curved, straight) blade, and it is used to lift up the _____ during intubation.

29. The MacIntosh blade is a _____ (curved, straight) blade, and its tip is placed in an area called the _____ during intubation.

30. The epiglottis _____ (is, is not) visible through the mouth when a straight blade is used, because the straight blade is placed under the epiglottis and _____ (part of the, the entire) soft tissue structure is lifted up anteriorly.

31. The tip of a curved blade rests at the vallecula, and it lifts the tongue only. Therefore, the epiglottis _____ (is, is not) visible through the mouth when a curved blade is used correctly.

32. During intubation, a _____ (straight, curved) blade lifts the tongue and epiglottis upward to expose the vocal cord and related structures, whereas a _____ (straight, curved) blade lifts the tongue only.

33. A _____ (straight, curved) blade functions better in patients with short necks, high or rigid larynxes, or obesity.

34. The tip of a curved blade can be positioned at the vallecula by advancing the tip of the curve blade to the base of the _____.

35. ET tubes come in sizes ranging from _____ to _____, and each size refers to the _____ (internal, external) diameter of the tube in millimeters (mm).

36. What is the purpose of the radiopaque line implanted along the length of an ET tube?

_____

_____

37. When intubating a spontaneously breathing patient, the ET tube is advanced into the trachea during _____ (inspiratory, expiratory) efforts when the vocal cords are open.

38. A syringe with a capacity of _____ mL or larger is used to test the pilot balloon before intubation and to inflate the cuff immediately after intubation.

39. After successful intubation, the cuff of an ET tube is inflated to _____ (provide ventilation, prevent air leak, apply pressure on the tracheal wall).

40. A(n) _____ (oil-based, water-soluble, petroleum-based) lubricant is used to lubricate the distal end of the ET tube for easy insertion into the trachea.

41. List two adverse outcomes that may occur if the ET tube is not secured properly.

_____

_____

42. A flexible stylet may be placed inside an ET tube to provide rigidity during oral and nasal intubation. _____ (TRUE/FALSE)

43. Magill forceps are used to perform _____ (oral intubation, nasal intubation, oral or nasal intubation, tracheotomy).

42 to 45. Match the patients with the estimated size of ET tubes. Use *only four* of the answers provided.

PATIENT	ESTIMATED SIZE
44. _____ 800-g neonate	A. 1 mm I.D.
45. _____ 4000-g neonate	B. 2.5 mm I.D.
46. _____ 8-year-old child	C. 4.0 mm I.D.
47. _____ Adult male	D. 5.0 mm I.D.
	E. 6.5 mm I.D.
	F. 8.0 mm I.D.

48. Given: Estimated ET tube size = 4.5 + (age/4). For a 10-year-old child, the estimated ET tube size should be:

   A. 5.

   B. 6.

   C. 7.

   D. 8.

49. During an intubation attempt, the pulse oximetry (SpO$_2$) reading drops from 95% to 83%, and the cardiac monitor shows persistent arrhythmias. This condition is most likely caused by:

   A. excessive ET tube size.

   B. prolonged intubation attempt.

   C. incorrect head position.

   D. cardiac arrest.

50. When a patient develops severe hypoxia and arrhythmias during an oral intubation attempt, all of the following steps should be done *except*:

   A. remove blade and ET tube from mouth.

   B. provide ventilation.

   C. provide oxygenation.

   D. use Magill forceps.

51. During oral intubation, the laryngoscope handle and blade should be _____ (pried against the upper teeth, lifted anteriorly to the patient) to clear the tongue and attached soft tissues.

52. Immediately after intubation, bilateral breath sounds are checked _____ (before, after) inflating the ET tube cuff.

53. Immediately after intubating an adult with a size 7 tube, the initial depth of insertion should be about _____ (18 cm, 22 cm, 26 cm) at the lips or incisors.

54. During nasal intubation, the ET tube is inserted through the nostril and then guided by the _____ (hemostat, fingers, Magill forceps) into the trachea.

55. Immediately after nasal intubation of a female adult with a size 7 tube, the initial depth of insertion should be about _____ (22 cm, 26 cm, 28 cm).

56. "Blind" nasal intubation is done by inserting the ET tube into the _____ (mouth, nostril) and advancing it slowly during spontaneous _____ (inspiratory, expiratory) efforts. When air movement is heard through the ET tube, it indicates that the distal end of the ET tube is near the _____ (esophagus, trachea).

57. Immediately after intubation, correct placement of the ET tube should be confirmed by verifying presence of bilateral breath sounds and:

    A. distance marking on the ET tube.

    B. chest radiograph.

    C. lateral neck radiograph.

    D. bowel sounds.

58. Esophageal intubation is a(n) _____ (insignificant, grave) error as it can lead to immediate _____ (pneumothorax, cardiac arrest, aspiration). This problem can be avoided by making sure that the ET tube passes through the _____ (area below the tongue, vocal cords, larynx) under direct vision.

59. Indications of successful and proper placement of an ET tube include all of the following *except*:

    A. presence of bilateral breath sounds.

    B. presence of CO_2 in expired gas.

    C. presence of condensations on the inside of ET tube during exhalation.

    D. presence of vocal sounds.

60. Bilateral breath sounds should be checked by placing the stethoscope diaphragm along the _____ (anterior aspect of the chest, midaxillary line).

61. Breath sounds should not be checked at the anterior chest locations close to the trachea, since airflow in the esophagus (i.e., in esophageal intubation) can give false "breath sounds" in neonates and thin adults. _____ (TRUE/FALSE)

62. In the absence of obvious lung pathology (e.g., atelectasis, consolidation, pleural effusion), uneven bilateral breath sounds may suggest _____ (esophageal, main-stem) intubation.

63. For adult patients, the tip of an ET tube should be about _____ (0.5, 1.5, 3) in. _____ (above, below) the carina.

64. Which of the following is *not* an adverse effect of unrecognized esophageal intubation?

    A. Hyperventilation

    B. Tissue and cerebral hypoxia

    C. Vomiting

    D. Aspiration

65. If the vocal cords are not seen or cannot be identified during intubation, the ET tube _____ (may be, should not be) inserted.

66. When the endotracheal tube is placed correctly into the tracheal, the collapsed esophageal bulb) should _____ (reinflate within 10 seconds, remain deflated after 10 seconds.

RAPID SEQUENCE INTUBATION

67. The primary reasons for rapid sequence intubation (RSI) is to optimize the intubation _____ (equipment and supplies, conditions), to protect the airway against _____ (rupture, aspiration), and to facilitate _____ (suctioning, ventilation and oxygenation).

68. A Glasgow coma scale of _____ (8 or higher, 8 or less) suggests severe brain injury and poor prognosis.

69. One of the indications for RSI is _____ (mild, moderate, severe) hypoxemia — a PaO_2/F_IO_2 (P/F) ratio of _____ (<250 mm Hg, >250 mm Hg).

70. RSI _____ (may, should not) be performed if a patient is able to sustain adequate ventilation and oxygenation while breathing spontaneously with other airways such as an oropharyngeal airway and laryngeal mask airway.

71. Etomidate (Amidate) is used for _____ (neuromuscular blockade, sedation, pain control) in RSI.

72. For adult patients, _____ (2, 20, 200) mg of etomidate may be given intravenously over _____ (1 to 10 sec, 30 to 60 sec) prior to RSI.

73. Succinylcholine is used to provide _____ (neuromuscular blockade, sedation, pain control) in RSI because it has rapid onset and _____ (long, short) duration of action.

74. The adult dosage of succinylcholine is about _____ mg or _____ mg/kg.

75. The onset of etomidate and succinylcholine is about _____ (10 sec, 60 sec, 3 min). Intubation supplies should be _____ (put together after, ready for use before) giving these drugs.

76. _____ (Sellick's, Heimlich, Jaw thrust) maneuver provides cricoid pressure to close off the _____ (trachea, esophagus) and to minimize aspiration.

77. The following drugs may be used if post-RSI paralysis and sedation are desired: vecuronium — a _____ (depolarizing, nondepolarizing) neuromuscular blocking agent); diazepam — an _____ (antianxiety, antibiotic) agent; and fentanyl — a _____ (natural, synthetic) opiate analgesic.

78. The suggested adult IV dosages for vecuronium, diazepam, and fentanyl are 0.1 mg/kg, 5–10 mg, and 200 µg, respectively. _____ (TRUE/FALSE)

MANAGEMENT OF ENDOTRACHEAL AND TRACHEOSTOMY TUBES

79. _____ (Endotracheal, Tracheostomy) tubes are secured by using adhesive tape or harness, and the _____ (endotracheal, tracheostomy) tubes are secured by a string around the neck which is tied to the two openings on the collar of the device.

80. Since the estimated capillary perfusion pressure in the trachea is about _____ (10 to 20, 25 to 35, 30 to 40) mm Hg, the *maximum* ET tube cuff pressure should not exceed _____ (10, 25, 30) mm Hg to allow adequate capillary perfusion in the trachea. For patients with _____ (hypertension, hypotension), the cuff pressure should be kept even lower to compensate for the _____ (increased, reduced) capillary flow.

81. Cuff pressure that is _____ (greater, less) than the capillary perfusion pressure in the trachea may cause ischemic injury and tissue necrosis.

82. The _____ (minimal leak technique, minimal occlusion volume) is obtained by slowly _____ (inflating, deflating) the cuff to a point at which no air leak is heard at _____ (end-inspiration, end-expiration) of a mechanical breath.

83. The _____ (end-inspiration, end-expiration) point is used during the minimal occlusion volume procedure because the trachea reaches its maximal size (diameter) at this point.

84. The _____ (minimal leak technique, minimal occlusion volume) is done by _____ (inflating, deflating) the cuff until the leak stops and then gradually removing a small amount of air until a *slight* leak can be heard at _____ (end-inspiration, end-expiration).

85. ET suctioning should be done regularly and frequently because it seldom causes mucosal damage, suction-induced hypoxemia, and arrhythmias. _____ (TRUE/FALSE)

86. The appropriate suction catheter size in French (Fr) may be estimated by multiplying the ET tube size in millimeter (mm) by _____ (2, 3), and then dividing by _____ (2, 3). The equation is Fr = (mm × 3)/2.

87. For endotracheal suctioning, the vacuum pressure should be kept between _____ (70 and 150, 100 and 200) mm Hg for adults and lower for infants and children. The optimal vacuum pressure for most adult patients is about _____ (100, 150, 200) mm Hg.

88. The duration of endotracheal suctioning for each attempt should be kept from _____ (1 to 5, 10 to 15, 15 to 30) sec for adults and no more than _____ (1, 5, 10) sec for pediatric patients.

89. The closed inline suction system helps to reduce suction-induced hypoxemia, because the ventilator circuit is not disconnected and the system maintains all ventilator settings such as F_IO_2 and PEEP. _____ (TRUE/FALSE)

90. ET tubes with dorsal lumen above the cuff are used to _____ (reduce the vacuum required for suctioning, remove secretions accumulated above the cuff).

91. The main steps of using the endotracheal tube changer involve inserting the tube changer into the existing ET tube, _____ (keeping the cuff inflated, deflating the cuff), stabilizing the changer and ET tube while removing the ET tube, replacing it with another ET tube, and inflating the cuff.

92. A fenestrated tracheostomy tube _____ (has, does not have) one or more openings along the body of the tube.

93. The patient may phonate or talk when the fenestrated tracheostomy tube opening _____ (remains open, is blocked) and the fenestration openings are _____ (open, closed).

94. A speaking valve is a _____ (one-way, two-way) valve put on a tracheostomy tube that allows the patient to breathe _____ (in and out, in only).

95. A speaking valve _____ (allows, blocks) the exhaled air from going through the tracheostomy tube opening and _____ (directs, blocks) the air through the vocal cords.

96. Contraindications for using a speaking valve include laryngeal stenosis, vocal cord paralysis, and severe tracheal stenosis. _____ (TRUE/FALSE)

97. When a speaking valve is used on a traditional tracheostomy tube, the cuff must be _____ (inflated, deflated).

98. When a speaking valve is used on a fenestrated tracheostomy tube, the fenestration openings must be _____ (open, closed).

99. When the speaking valve is placed on a fenestrated tracheostomy tube with a nonfenestrated inner cannula, the inner cannula must be _____ (kept in place, removed).

100. A speaking valve is intended for users who are breathing spontaneously, and it must not be used during mechanical ventilation. _____ (TRUE/FALSE)

EXTUBATION

101. In addition to blood gases, muscle strengths, and general cardiopulmonary signs, the rapid shallow breathing index can be a useful indicator of readiness for extubation. It is calculated by: (f = frequency, V_T = spontaneous tidal volume)

    A. $f + V_T$

    B. $f - V_T$

    C. $f \times V_T$

    D. f/V_T

102. A rapid shallow breathing index of _____ (more, less) than 100 breaths/min/L (or cycles/L) is highly predictive of a successful extubation outcome.

103. The f and V_T measurements should be collected as soon as the patient is taken off ventilatory support and begins breathing spontaneously. _____ (TRUE/FALSE)

104. Other criteria that are useful for predicting a successful extubation outcome include: spontaneous minute ventilation less than _____ L/min with satisfactory oxygenation, PaO_2/F_IO_2 (P/F ratio) more than _____ mm Hg, maximal inspiratory pressure greater than _____ cm H_2O, vital capacity greater than _____ mL/kg, and absence of cardiopulmonary problems.

105. A 68-year-old COPD patient extubated himself inadvertently. The therapist has been asked to evaluate this patient for possible reintubation. Seven clinical predictors are available, and they are as follows: (1) SIMV rate = 10/min, (2) most recent pH = 7.33, (3) most recent PaO_2/F_IO_2 = 160 mm Hg, (4) highest heart rate in the past 24 hours = 130/min, (5) patient's diagnosis is COPD, CHF, and renal failure, (6) patient is alert, and (7) patient is on ventilator due to ventilatory failure.

    Referring to the data provided above select the best set of answers to complete the following statement:

    Based on the clinical predictors for reintubation, the therapist should recommend that the patient _____ since he has met _____ of the predictors.

    A. be reintubated, 3

    B. be reintubated, 5

    C. not be reintubated, 3

    D. not be reintubated, 5

COMPLICATIONS OF ENDOTRACHEAL AIRWAY

106. Which of the following is *not* a potential complication during intubation?

    A. Trauma to teeth and soft tissues

    B. Hoarseness

    C. Vomiting and aspiration

    D. Hypoxia and arrhythmias

107. The ASA Task Force on the Management of the Difficult Airway recommends a limit of _____ (three, five, seven) intubation attempts to minimize patient injury.

108. Which of the following is *not* a potential complication while the patient is intubated?

    A. Loss of coughing reflex

    B. Aspiration from feeding

    C. Main-stem intubation

    D. Inadvertent extubation

109. Which of the following is *not* a potential complication immediately after extubation?

    A. Aspiration

    B. Laryngospasm

    C. Vomiting

    D. Laryngeal and subglottic edema

110. Which of the following is *not* a potential long-term complication some time after extubation?

    A. Trauma to teeth and soft tissues

    B. Laryngeal stenosis

    C. Tracheal inflammation, dilation, and stenosis

    D. Vocal cord paralysis

111. Esophageal intubation is more likely committed by inexperienced practitioners. _____ (TRUE/FALSE)

112. Excessive stimulation of the _____ (phrenic, vagus, medial supraclavicular) nerve during intubation attempt can cause bradycardia.

113. While the patient is intubated, kinking of an ET tube leads to _____ (high, low) peak inspiratory pressure and _____ (increased, reduced) airflow.

114. For an orally intubated patient, the distance marking on the ET tube (e.g., 22 cm) is the distance from the distal end of the ET tube to the patient's _____ (lips or incisors, nares).

115. Extubation should be done when the patient is either deeply anesthetized, or, preferably, semiconscious, because laryngospasm usually occurs when the patient is fully awake. _____ (TRUE/FALSE)

116. Stridor is the _____ (harsh or high-pitched sound, gentle or low-pitched sound) heard during spontaneous breathing. It is heard when the upper airway is _____ (partially, completely) obstructed.

117. Mild stridor following extubation is initially treated with _____ aerosolized (epinephrine, racemic epinephrine).

CHAPTER 7

Noninvasive Positive Pressure Ventilation

TERMINOLOGY

1. Noninvasive positive pressure ventilation (NPPV) refers to a mechanical ventilation strategy without a(n) _____ .

2. Continuous positive airway pressure (CPAP) _____ (does, does not) include mechanical breaths, and the work of breathing is entirely assumed by the _____ (ventilator, patient).

3. Bilevel positive airway pressure (bilevel PAP) can be used to provide _____ (one, two, one or two) level(s) of airway pressure.

4. When bilevel PAP is used, the peak inspiratory pressure is controlled by the _____ (IPAP, EPAP) setting, and the CPAP or PEEP level is controlled by the _____ (IPAP, EPAP) setting.

PHYSIOLOGIC EFFECTS OF NPPV

5. If a larger tidal volume is desired, the _____ (IPAP, EPAP) level is typically _____ (increased, decreased) to increase the pressure gradient between IPAP and EPAP.

6. The functional residual capacity can be increased by increasing the _____ (IPAP, EPAP) level.

7. _____ (IPAP, EPAP) relieves upper airway obstruction with its splinting action.

8. List two or more laboratory parameters that may be used as titration endpoints for the appropriate initial IPAP and EPAP levels.

   _____

   _____

   _____

USE OF CONTINUOUS POSITIVE AIRWAY PRESSURE

9. CPAP provides positive airway pressure during the _____ (inspiratory phase, expiratory phase, entire spontaneous breath), and it _____ (does, does not) include any mechanical breaths.

10. Compared to mechanical ventilation, CPAP imposes _____ (more, less) work of breathing on the patient.

11. CPAP is considered a noninvasive ventilation strategy because it _____ (does, does not) typically require an artificial airway.

12. When the inspiratory pressure and expiratory pressure of a bilevel PAP device are set at the same level, _____ (IPPB, CPAP, PEEP) results.

13. CPAP is the treatment of choice for _____ (central, obstructive, mixed) sleep apnea without significant carbon dioxide retention.

14. CPAP should *not* be used to manage apnea that is due to _____ (airflow obstruction, neuromuscular causes).

15. Sleep apnea is defined as a temporary pause in breathing that lasts at least _____ (5, 10, 20) sec during sleep.

16. The cause of obstructive sleep apnea is severe _____ (lung volume restriction, airflow obstruction) during sleep.

17. If a patient sleeps for 6 hours and has 120 apnea episodes. The _____ (apnea index, apnea-hypopnea index, desaturation index) would be 20.

18. Hypopnea is defined as reduction of airflow to _____ (≥25%, ≥50%, ≥70%) of the baseline amplitude for _____ (5, 10, 30) seconds. This condition is usually associated with a reduction of oxygen saturation by _____ (≥2%, ≥4%, ≥8%) of the patient's baseline value.

19. Hypopnea is associated with oxygen desaturation and pulse alteration. _____ (TRUE/FALSE)

20. The apnea-hypopnea index is the number of:

    A. apneas and hypopneas per hour of sleep.

    B. apneas and hypopneas during test.

    C. apneas during test/number of hypopneas during test.

    D. apneas and hypopneas in 8 hours of sleep.

21. Which of the following is *not* a risk factor for obstructive sleep apnea?

    A. Obesity

    B. Increased neck circumference

    C. Hypertension

    D. History of smoking

22. Prosthetic mandibular advancement, tonsillectomy, uvulopalatopharyngoplasty, weight reduction gastric surgery, and CPAP are some strategies for the management of _____ (central sleep apnea, obstructive sleep apnea, mixed apnea).

USE OF BILEVEL POSITIVE AIRWAY PRESSURE

23. Bilevel PAP has an inspiratory positive airway pressure (IPAP) setting that provides _____ (ventilation, oxygenation) and an expiratory positive airway pressure (EPAP) level that functions as _____ (positive end-expiratory pressure, pressure support).

24. List two major indications for bilevel PAP when it is used as an adjunct to provide mechanical ventilation.

    _____

    _____

25. For patients with hypoxemic respiratory failure, refractory hypoxemia is present when the PaO_2/F_IO_2 (P/F) ratio is _____ (more than, less than) 250 mm Hg.

26. Which of the following is *not* an indication for NPPV?

    A. Reduction of respiratory workload in obesity

    B. Acute respiratory failure

    C. Noncardiogenic pulmonary edema

    D. Acute hypercapnic exacerbations of COPD

27. Contraindications for NPPV include all of the following *except*:

    A. apnea.

    B. inability to handle secretions.

    C. facial trauma.

    D. exacerbations of COPD.

28. Patients who are unable to handle secretions should not be placed on NPPV because _____ (hypoventilation, aspiration, respiratory failure, apnea) can be a potential problem without an artificial airway.

COMMON INTERFACES FOR CPAP AND BILEVEL PAP

29. In NPPV, the external device that connects the ventilator tubing to the patient's nose, mouth, or face is called a(n) _____.

30. List four interfaces used in NPPV.

    _____

    _____

    _____

    _____

31. When a nasal mask is used during NPPV, it _____ (must have a tight seal, may have a minor leak, should have a large leak).

32. In selecting a new nasal mask, a common error is selecting one that is too _____ (large, small) for the patient.

33. If air leak around the nasal mask is significant after trying on different sizes, the _____ (Nasal Pillows™, oronasal mask, endotracheal tube, laryngeal mask airway) should be considered.

34. Another problem with a nasal mask is air leak through the _____, particularly when the positive pressure level is high.

35. Immediately after setting up the nasal mask, _____ (pulse oximetry, blood gas analysis) is done to check for improvement in oxygenation. This should be followed by _____ (pulse oximetry, blood gas analysis) for fine-tuning the pressure settings.

36. List two advantages of using a nasal mask during NPPV.

   _____

   _____

37. List two disadvantages of using a nasal mask during NPPV.

   _____

   _____

38. _____ (An oronasal mask, Nasal Pillows™) is an interface used in NPPV that covers the patient's nose and mouth area.

39. Since an oronasal mask covers the patient's nose and mouth, list two potentially harmful problems in using this interface.

   _____

   _____

40. Besides regurgitation, aspiration, and asphyxiation, list three disadvantages of using an oronasal mask during NPPV.

   _____

   _____

41. Nasal Pillows™ resembles a small nasal mask, and it consists of two small cushions that fit under the _____ . It is commonly used during _____ (bilevel PAP, CPAP, IPPB) therapy.

42. Since Nasal Pillows™ can withstand airway pressures of up to _____ (10, 20, 30, 40) cm H_2O, they are _____ (more, less) effective than the nasal and oronasal masks in the bilevel PAP mode.

43. A full-face mask does not inherit problems with air leaks and pressure sores around the nose and mouth because this mask _____ (does, does not) make contact with the nose and mouth.

44. The full-face mask is ideal for all of the following patients or conditions *except*:

    A. status asthmaticus.

    B. claustrophobic patients.

    C. mouth breathers.

    D. patients without teeth or with facial abnormalities.

POTENTIAL PROBLEMS WITH INTERFACES

45. Which of the following should not be done to reduce air leaks through an interface during NPPV?

    A. Adjusting headgear and use chin strap

    B. Trying another size or mask

    C. Reducing pressure setting

    D. Using spacers or foam pads

46. Which of the following is not effective in minimizing skin breakdown or irritation during NPPV?

    A. Adjusting or trying another headgear

    B. Using chin strap

    C. Using spacers, foam pads, or topical ointments

    D. Trying a different cleaning solution

TITRATION OF CONTINUOUS POSITIVE AIRWAY PRESSURE

47. The *initial* CPAP setting should be _____ (2, 4, 6, 8) cm H_2O.

48. If the bilevel PAP device does not have a separate CPAP control, a CPAP level of 4 cm H_2O may be obtained by setting the:

    A. IPAP at 4 cm H_2O and EPAP at 0 cm H_2O.

    B. IPAP at 8 cm H_2O and EPAP at 4 cm H_2O.

    C. IPAP and EPAP at 4 cm H_2O.

    D. IPAP at 0 cm H_2O and EPAP at 4 cm H_2O.

49. The appropriate CPAP level for a patient with sleep apnea is titrated by observing the following parameters:

    A. SpO_2 readings and number of apnea episodes.

    B. number of apnea episodes.

    C. PCO_2 and SpO_2 readings.

    D. PO_2 and SpO_2 readings.

50. _____ (Ramp, Autotitration, C-Flex™) is a strategy done by the CPAP machine to self-adjust the delivered airway pressure according to the patient's needs.

51. Ramp is a feature of the CPAP machine in which the starting pressure increases gradually, over a span of up to _____ (15 min, 45 min), until the desired pressure is reached.

52. C-Flex™ is a feature of the CPAP machine that provides pressure relief during _____ (inhalation, exhalation). This reduces the continuous pressure which the patient must overcome during _____ (inhalation, exhalation).

TITRATION OF BILEVEL POSITIVE AIRWAY PRESSURES

53. The *initial* bilevel PAP settings are typically IPAP at _____ (0, 4, 8, 12, 16) cm H_2O, and EPAP at _____ (0, 4, 8, 12, 16) cm H_2O.

54. The IPAP maximum time should be set at _____ (0.01 to 0.03, 0.15 to 0.25, 0.5 to 0.7) sec longer than the patient's actual inspiratory time, and the IPAP maximum time should not be longer than _____ (30%, 40%, 50%) of the respiratory cycle.

55. The IPAP level is increased in _____ cm H_2O increments to provide more _____.

56. The EPAP level is increased in _____ cm H_2O increments to _____.

57. If poor synchronization occurs during NPPV, check for _____ (air leaks, oxygen flow, pressure settings) or alter _____ (EPAP level, IPAP level, IPAP maximum time).

58. Oxygen should be added if the baseline oxygen saturation remains low with appropriate IPAP and EPAP settings. _____ (TRUE/FALSE)

59. IPAP or EPAP level should be set according to patient tolerance. _____ (TRUE/FALSE)

60. Bi-Flex™ is a feature of bilevel PAP in which _____ (1, 2, 3, 4) level(s) of adjustable pressure _____ (support, relief) is provided to the patient.

61. Bi-Flex™ is a feature of bilevel PAP in which pressure relief is provided to the patient at the end of _____ (inhalation, exhalation) and the start of _____ (inhalation, exhalation).

CHAPTER 8

Initiation of Mechanical Ventilation

GOALS OF MECHANICAL VENTILATION

1. Which of the following is *not* a goal of mechanical ventilation?

   A. Prevent lung infection

   B. Improve oxygenation and remove carbon dioxide

   C. Relieve excessive work of breathing

   D. Improve lung mechanics

INDICATIONS

2. Mechanical ventilation is indicated in all of the following conditions *except*:

   A. acute or impending ventilatory failure.

   B. severe hypoxemia.

   C. prophylatic ventilatory support.

   D. metabolic acid-base imbalance.

3. Acute ventilatory failure is defined as a _____ (gradual, sudden) increase of the _____ ($PaCO_2$, PaO_2) to greater than 50 mm Hg with an accompanying respiratory _____ (acidosis, alkalosis).

4. In patients with chronic CO_2 retention, mechanical ventilation may be indicated when the $PaCO_2$ is more than 10 mm Hg _____ (above, below) the patient's baseline value with an accompanying respiratory _____ (acidosis, alkalosis) and a pH generally _____ (more, less) than 7.30.

5. Impending ventilatory failure becomes evident when the _____ (pH, $PaCO_2$, PaO_2) shows a(n) _____ (acute, gradual and persistent) increase.

6. At the early stage of impending ventilatory failure, the $PaCO_2$ value may be normal or low due to _____ (renal, respiratory) compensation for the gas exchange deficiencies. This compensation is characterized by a temporary alveolar _____ (hyperventilation, hypoventilation).

7. Five clinical signs have been used to indicate the development of impending ventilatory failure. Complete the table below to define the threshold for each clinical sign.

CLINICAL SIGNS FOR IMPENDING VENTILATORY FAILURE	THRESHOLDS
_____ Spontaneous V_T	Less than _____ mL/kg
_____ Spontaneous frequency	_____ (Greater than, Less than) 25 to 35/min
_____ Spontaneous minute volume	Greater than _____ L
_____ Vital capacity	Less than _____ mL/kg
_____ Maximal inspiratory pressure	Less than _____ cm H_2O

8. Severe hypoxemia is present when the PaO_2 is less than _____ (60, 80) mm Hg on F_IO_2 of greater than _____ (30%, 50%) or the PaO_2 is less than _____ (40, 60) mm Hg at any F_IO_2.

9. When the $P(A\text{-}a)O_2$ measurement is used to evaluate a patient's oxygenation status, every 50 mm Hg difference in $P(A\text{-}a)O_2$ approximates _____ (2, 5, 10)% of intrapulmonary shunt (at an F_IO_2 of 100%).

10. Given: P_AO_2 = 260 mm Hg, PaO_2 = 70 mm Hg. What is the calculated $P(A\text{-}a)O_2$ and the estimated shunt percent?

   A. $P(A\text{-}a)O_2$ = 150 mm Hg, 3% shunt

   B. $P(A\text{-}a)O_2$ = 150 mm Hg, 6% shunt

   C. $P(A\text{-}a)O_2$ = 190 mm Hg, 6% shunt

   D. $P(A\text{-}a)O_2$ = 190 mm Hg, 8% shunt

11. The P_AO_2 can be calculated by using the alveolar air equation below.

   A. $P_AO_2 = (P_B - PH_2O) \times F_IO_2$

   B. $P_AO_2 = (P_B - PH_2O) \times F_IO_2 - PaCO_2$

   C. $P_AO_2 = (P_B - PH_2O) \times F_IO_2 - (PaCO_2/R)$

   D. $P_AO_2 = (P_B - PH_2O) \times F_IO_2 - (PaCO_2 \times 1.5)$

12. The PaO_2/F_IO_2 (P/F ratio) may be used to evaluate the degree of _____ (hypercapnia, hypoxemia) in patients with acute lung injury (ALI) or acute respiratory distress syndrome (ARDS).

13. For ALI, the PaO_2/F_IO_2 (P/F ratio) threshold is _____ ($\leq$ 200 mm Hg, $\leq$ 300 mm Hg). For ARDS, it is _____ ($\leq$ 200 mm Hg, $\leq$ 300 mm Hg).

14. Since ALI and ARDS also exhibit bilateral infiltrates, a PCWP value of _____ (higher than, lower than) 18 mm Hg is used to *rule out* bilateral infiltrates caused by cardiogenic pulmonary edema.

15. Acute onset of bilateral alveolar infiltrates along with a PCWP of $\leq$18 mm Hg is _____ (consistent, inconsistent) with ALI or ARDS.

16. Prophylatic ventilatory support is provided in clinical conditions in which the risk of pulmonary complications, ventilatory failure, or oxygenation failure is relatively low. _____ (TRUE/FALSE)

CONTRAINDICATIONS

17. Positive pressure ventilation is contraindicated in untreated:

A. pleural effusion.

B. hemothorax.

C. tension pneumothorax.

D. all of the above.

18. Positive pressure ventilation may be used to ventilate patients with tension pneumothorax after placement of a _____ to relieve the pleural _____ (fluid, blood, pressure).

19. Initiation of mechanical ventilation is sometimes withheld:

A. on patient's request.

B. in cases of medical futility.

C. to reduce or terminate a patient's pain and suffering.

D. all of the above.

20. Medical futility means that medical intervention is most likely to be _____ (useful, useless) based on previous experience in similar cases.

INITIAL VENTILATOR SETTINGS

21. _____ (Full, Partial) ventilatory support (i.e., control mode, assist/control mode, high synchronized intermittent mandatory ventilation [SIMV] frequency) is necessary if the patient is apneic.

22. Partial ventilatory support is indicated if the patient is _____ (able, unable) to assume _____ (part, all) of the work of breathing.

23. Dual control mode combines _____ (one, two, three) control variables that are regulated by the _____ (ventilator, patient).

24. The effectiveness of dual control mode is better than single control mode, and it has been thoroughly tested and validated with controlled clinical trials. _____ (TRUE/FALSE)

25. The initial ventilator frequency may be estimated to provide _____ (hyperventilation, eucapneic ventilation, hyperoxia).

26. Eucapneic ventilation is achieved when the patient's $PaCO_2$ is at _____ (40 mm Hg, the patient's normal value).

27. The initial ventilator frequency may be set between _____ (6 to 8, 10 to 12, 14 to 16) breaths per minute.

28. High frequency (e.g., 20 or more breaths/min) during mechanical ventilation may not allow adequate time for _____ (inhalation, exhalation). This, in turn, may lead to development of air trapping and _____ (hyperventilation, hypoventilation, auto-PEEP).

29. List three conditions that may lead to auto-PEEP.

_____

_____

_____

30. The ventilator frequency is the primary control to regulate a patient's _____ (pH, heart rate, PaO_2, $PaCO_2$).

31. In general, the frequency setting on a ventilator should be _____ (increased, decreased) if the $PaCO_2$ is too high; _____ (increased, decreased) if the $PaCO_2$ is too low.

32. The initial tidal volume setting on the ventilator should be set between _____ (6 to 10, 10 to 12, 12 to 15) mL/kg of predicted body weight.

33. Occasionally, tidal volumes as low as 6 mL/kg are used to provide intentional _____ (hyperventilation, hypoventilation). This type of ventilation (i.e., permissive hypercapnia) is done to minimize the airway pressures and the risk of _____ (hyperventilation, auto-PEEP, barotrauma).

34. Decreasing the tidal volume by 100 to 200 mL is one strategy used to _____ (increase, lessen) the expiratory time requirement so as to prevent _____ (atelectasis, hypoventilation, air trapping), particularly in patients with COPD.

35 to 37. Certain clinical conditions may benefit from lower ventilator tidal volumes for reducing airway pressures. Match the conditions below with the respective examples. Use each answer *once*.

CONDITION	EXAMPLE
35. _____ Increase of airway pressure requirement	A. Pneumonectomy
36. _____ Increase of lung compliance	B. ARDS
37. _____ Decrease of lung volumes	C. Emphysema

38. The tidal volume delivered to the patient by the ventilator is usually _____ (higher, lower) than the preset tidal volume, due to gas leakage and circuit compressible volume loss.

39. Given: Expired volume = 120 mL; PEEP = 0 cm H_2O. Peak inspiratory pressure with complete wye occlusion = 30 cm H_2O. Calculate the ventilator circuit compression factor.

    A. 2 mL/cm H_2O

    B. 3 mL/cm H_2O

    C. 4 mL/cm H_2O

    D. 5 mL/cm H_2O

40. Given: Circuit compression factor = 3 mL/cm H_2O; peak inspiratory pressure (PIP) during mechanical ventilation = 50 cm H_2O; PEEP = 10 cm H_2O. Calculate the circuit compression volume (lost volume) at these pressure readings.

    A. 17 mL

    B. 60 mL

    C. 120 mL

    D. 150 mL

41. Given: Expired tidal volume = 700 mL; circuit compression volume = 120 mL. What is the corrected tidal volume?

    A. 480 mL

    B. 580 mL

    C. 720 mL

    D. 820 mL

42. Pressure support ventilation (PSV) is used to augment a patient's breathing effort by reducing the airflow resistance during _____ (mechanical ventilation, spontaneous breathing).

43. Pressure support (PS) is available only in modes of ventilation that allows spontaneous breathing. _____ (TRUE/FALSE)

44. To calculate the initial pressure support level, all of the following ventilator and patient parameters are required *except*:

    A. peak inspiratory pressure.

    B. positive end-expiratory pressure.

    C. plateau pressure.

    D. inspiratory flows of ventilator and patient.

45. For *weaning* from mechanical ventilation with a *spontaneous breathing trial*, PS is titrated until achieving a spontaneous frequency of _____ (10 to 15, 20 to 25, 30 to 40) breaths/min or a spontaneous tidal volume of _____ (4 to 6, 8 to 10, 12 to 14) ml/kg predicted body weight (PBW).

46. The PS level is reduced by _____ (1 to 2, 2 to 4, 4 to 6) cm H_2O increments during the weaning process.

47. For patients with severe hypoxemia, the initial F_IO_2 may be set at 100%. It should be adjusted until the _____ (PaO_2, $PaCO_2$) is maintained between _____ (80 and 100 mm Hg, 35 and 45 mm Hg) for normal patients but _____ (higher, lower) for patients with chronic CO_2 retention.

48. After the patient has been stabilized, the F_IO_2 should be kept below _____ (30%, 50%, 70%) to avoid oxygen-induced lung injuries.

49. For patients with mild hypoxemia or normal cardiopulmonary functions (e.g., drug overdose, uncomplicated postoperative recovery), the initial F_IO_2 may be set at _____ or at the patient's F_IO_2 prior to mechanical ventilation.

50. For patients with refractory hypoxemia, the initial PEEP level may be set at _____ cm H_2O. Subsequent changes of PEEP should be based on the patient's blood gas results, F_IO_2 requirement, tolerance of PEEP, and cardiovascular responses.

51. The initial I:E ratio is usually kept in a range between _____ and _____. A larger I:E ratio (longer E ratio) may be used on patients needing additional time for exhalation because of the possibility of _____ (atelectasis, air trapping) and auto-PEEP.

52. Presence of air trapping during mechanical ventilation may be checked by occluding the _____ (inspiratory, expiratory) port of the ventilator circuit at the _____ (beginning, end) of exhalation. Auto-PEEP is present when the _____ (beginning-expiratory pressure, end-expiratory pressure) does not return to the baseline pressure.

53. Inverse I:E ratio has been used to correct refractory hypoxemia in ARDS patients with very _____ (high, low) lung compliance.

54. In addition to the inspiratory flow rate (peak flow), all of the following ventilator controls may affect the I:E ratio *except*:

    A. frequency.

    B. inspiratory time or inspiratory time %.

    C. minute volume.

    D. positive end-expiratory pressure.

55. By increasing the inspiratory flow rate (peak flow), the inspiratory time (I time) becomes _____ (longer, shorter) and the expiratory time (E time) becomes _____ (longer, shorter). [Assume the V_T and f are unchanged.]

56. Describe the effects of decreasing the inspiratory flow on the I time and E time. [Assume the V_T and f are kept unchanged.]

_____

_____

57. By increasing the tidal volume, the I time becomes _____ (longer, shorter) and the E time becomes _____ (longer, shorter). [Assume the flow rate and f are unchanged.]

58. Describe the effects of lowering the tidal volume on the I time and E time. [Assume the flow rate and f are kept unchanged.]

_____

_____

59. When the flow rate and V_T are kept constant, changes in the f have little effect on the _____ (I time, E time), but the _____ (I time, E time) is affected greatly by the frequency.

60. A higher f _____ (lengthens, shortens) the E time and a slower f _____ (lengthens, shortens) the E time. [Assume the flow rate and V_T are kept unchanged.]

61. Given: Minute volume = 12 L/min. Calculate the minimum flow rate needed for an I:E ratio of 1:4.

    A. 30 L/min

    B. 40 L/min

    C. 50 L/min

    D. 60 L/min

62. Given: f = 12/min. Calculate the I time and E time needed for an I:E ratio of 1:3.

    A. I time = 0.75 sec; E time = 4.25 sec

    B. I time = 1 sec; E time = 4 sec

    C. I time = 1.25 sec; E time = 3.75 sec

    D. I time = 1.5 sec; E time = 3.5 sec

63. Given: Calculate the I time % needed for an I:E ratio of 1:3.

    A. 25%

    B. 33%

    C. 50%

    D. 67%

64. List the four common flow patterns available on adult ventilators.

    _____

    _____

65. Selection of a flow pattern on the ventilator should be based on the patient's condition and the measurable improvement of the patient's ventilatory and oxygenation status on a selected flow pattern. _____ (TRUE/FALSE)

VENTILATOR ALARM SETTINGS

66. The low exhaled volume alarm (low volume alarm) is typically used to detect _____ (excessive system pressure, system leak) or _____ (circuit obstruction, circuit disconnection).

67. The low exhaled volume alarm should be set at about _____ (100 mL, 200 mL, 300 mL) _____ (higher, lower) than the _____ (preset, expired) mechanical tidal volume.

68. The low inspiratory pressure alarm is used to detect system leak or circuit disconnection. _____ (TRUE/FALSE)

69. The low inspiratory pressure alarm should be set at _____ (0 to 10 cm H_2O, 10 to 15 cm H_2O, 15 to 20 cm H_2O) _____ (above, below) the observed PIP.

70. The high inspiratory pressure alarm (high pressure limit alarm) should be set at _____ (0 to 10 cm H_2O, 10 to 15 cm H_2O, 15 to 20 cm H_2O) _____ (above, below) the observed PIP.

71. The high inspiratory pressure alarm may be triggered by all of the following conditions *except*:

    A. secretions in the airway.

    B. kinking or biting of the endotracheal tube.

    C. bronchospasm.

    D. circuit disconnection.

72. Once the high inspiratory pressure is triggered, _____ (inspiration, expiration) is immediately terminated and the ventilator goes to the _____ (inspiratory, expiratory) cycle. As a result, the volume delivered by the ventilator will become _____ (larger, smaller).

73. The apnea alarm is triggered by:

    A. apnea.

    B. circuit disconnection.

    C. cuff deflation.

    D. all of the above.

74. The apnea alarm should be set with a _____ (1 to 10 sec, 15 to 20 sec, 25 to 40 sec) time delay.

75. The high frequency alarm should be set at _____ (1 to 10 breaths/min, 10 to 15 breaths/min, 25 to 40 breaths/min) _____ (over, below) the observed frequency.

76. Triggering of the high frequency alarm is a sign of _____ (alveolar hyperventilation, alveolar hypoventilation, respiratory distress).

77. The high F_IO_2 alarm should be set at 5 to 10% _____ (over, below) the analyzed F_IO_2, and the low F_IO_2 alarm should be set at 5 to 10% _____ (over, below) the analyzed F_IO_2.

78 to 84. Match the given ventilator parameters with the initial alarm settings. Choose *one* answer from each set of answers provided.

78. Given: Expired volume = 700 mL

    A. Low volume alarm = 500 mL

    B. Low volume alarm = 600 mL

    C. Low volume alarm = 800 mL

    D. Low volume alarm = 900 mL

79. Given: PIP = 60 cm H_2O

    A. Low pressure alarm = 45 cm H_2O

    B. Low pressure alarm = 55 cm H_2O

    C. Low pressure alarm = 65 cm H_2O

    D. Low pressure alarm = 75 cm H_2O

80. Given: PIP = 45 cm H_2O

    A. High pressure alarm = 35 cm H_2O

    B. High pressure alarm = 45 cm H_2O

    C. High pressure alarm = 50 cm H_2O

    D. High pressure alarm = 60 cm H_2O

81. Given: Ventilator SIMV frequency = 8/min

    A. Apnea time delay = 5 sec

    B. Apnea time delay = 10 sec

    C. Apnea time delay = 20 sec

    D. Apnea time delay = 30 sec

82. Given: Ventilator SIMV frequency = 8/min

    A. High frequency alarm = 10/min

    B. High frequency alarm = 20/min

    C. High frequency alarm = 30/min

    D. High frequency alarm = 40/min

83. Given: Analyzed F_IO_2 = 50%

    A. High F_IO_2 alarm = 35%

    B. High F_IO_2 alarm = 45%

    C. High F_IO_2 alarm = 55%

    D. High F_IO_2 alarm = 65%

84. Given: Analyzed F_IO_2 = 50%

    A. Low F_IO_2 alarm = 35%

    B. Low F_IO_2 alarm = 45%

    C. Low F_IO_2 alarm = 55%

    D. Low F_IO_2 alarm = 65%

HAZARDS AND COMPLICATIONS

85 to 88. Match the conditions leading to complications in mechanical ventilation with the respective examples. Use each answer *once*.

	CONDITION	EXAMPLE
85. _____	Related to positive pressure ventilation	A. Nosocomial pneumonia
86. _____	Related to patient condition	B. Physical and psychologic trauma
87. _____	Related to ventilator supplies	C. Barotrauma
88. _____	Related to medical professionals	D. Circuit disconnection

89. Ventilator alarms are essentially foolproof, and they rarely require preventive maintenance and testing. _____ (TRUE/FALSE)

90. Barotrauma is lung tissue injury or rupture that is primarily caused by the shearing force of alveolar _____ (atelectasis, overdistention).

91. Risk of barotrauma may be increased when the airway pressures are higher than normal. Complete the table below to state the thresholds that may increase the likelihood of barotrauma.

AIRWAY PRESSURES RELATED TO BAROTRAUMA	THRESHOLDS
_____ PIP	Greater than _____ cm H_2O
_____ Plateau pressure	Greater than _____ cm H_2O
_____ Mean airway pressure	Greater than _____ cm H_2O
_____ PEEP	Greater than _____ cm H_2O

92. During mechanical ventilation, development of barotrauma is _____ (more, less) likely in COPD patients due to _____ (fibrosis, air trapping) and _____ (tightened, weakened) lung tissues.

93. Other lung injuries that may occur as a result of positive pressure ventilation include all of the following *except*:

    A. pulmonary interstitial emphysema.

    B. pulmonary fibrosis.

    C. pneumomediastinum.

    D. subcutaneous emphysema.

94. Since positive pressure ventilation compresses the pulmonary arterial vessels, the blood is backed up into the right atrium. This condition _____ (increases, decreases) the central venous pressure. The pressure gradient between the right atrium and the systemic venous drainage will therefore be _____ (increased, decreased).

95. A reduced pressure gradient between the right atrium and the venous drainage means a _____ (higher, lower) venous return to the right atrium and _____ (higher, lower) cardiac output.

96. In patients with a competent cardiovascular system, a small drop in venous return may be compensated by _____ (increasing, decreasing) the heart rate and _____ (constricting, dilating) the arterial blood vessels.

97. High airway pressures are more detrimental to the cardiac output in patients with _____ (high, low) lung compliance than those with _____ (high, low) compliance, due to the dampening effects of low lung compliance.

CHAPTER 9

Monitoring in Mechanical Ventilation

VITAL SIGNS

1. The normal adult heart rate is between _____ and _____ per minute.

2. Tachycardia means a heart rate greater than _____.

3. Tachycardia may be caused by all of the following clinical conditions *except*:

    A. hypoxemia.

    B. hypovolemia.

    C. fever.

    D. hypothermia.

4. Bradycardia means a heart rate less than _____.

5. Bradycardia may be caused by all of the following clinical conditions *except*:

    A. pain and stress.

    B. sinoatrial node malfunction.

    C. obstruction of coronary blood flow.

    D. prolonged suctioning.

6. A patient's blood pressure may be monitored via an indwelling arterial catheter inserted in any of the following arteries *except* the:

    A. brachial artery.

    B. popliteal artery.

    C. carotid artery.

    D. radial artery.

7. Fluid overload, vasoconstriction, stress, anxiety, and pain may initially lead to _____ (hypertension, hypotension, cardiac arrest).

8. When hypotension occurs during positive pressure ventilation, it is often associated with _____ (excessive, inadequate) intrathoracic pressure, peak inspiratory pressure, and lung volume.

9. Absolute hypovolemia can lead to _____ (hypertension, hypotension). An example of *absolute* hypovolemia is _____ (hemorrhage, shock).

10. Relative hypovolemia can also lead to _____ (hypertension, hypotension). An example of *relative* hypovolemia is _____ (dehydration, sepsis).

11. In general, absolute hypovolemia is related to _____ (excessive, inadequate) circulating volume, and it can be corrected by blood or fluid replacement.

12. Relative hypovolemia is related to _____ (excessive, loss of) venous tone. When the venous vessels dilate, the relative amount of circulating volume becomes _____ (excessive, inadequate). Relative hypovolemia can be corrected by treating the cause of venous dilation and *partial* fluid replacement.

13. Hypervolemia and positive pressure ventilation are two causes of hypotension. _____ (TRUE/FALSE)

14. The normal spontaneous respiratory frequency for adults is _____ breaths per minute.

15. Tachypnea means a(n) _____ (increased, decreased) respiratory frequency, and it may be an early warning sign of _____ (respiratory alkalosis, respiratory distress).

16. One strategy of weaning from mechanical ventilation is to allow the patient to breathe spontaneously without ventilator assistance. When tachypnea and low tidal volume are observed in a spontaneously breathing patient, it is indicative of _____ (successful, unsuccessful) weaning outcome.

17. _____ (Hyperthermia, Hypothermia) may be caused by conditions that increase a patient's metabolic rate and oxygen utilization. Furthermore, it shifts the oxyhemoglobin dissociation curve to the _____ (right, left), causing a _____ (higher, lower) oxygen saturation at any PaO_2.

18. Hypothermia is *least* likely caused by:

    A. infection.

    B. central nervous system (CNS) problem.

    C. metabolic disorder.

    D. cold exposure.

19. _____ (Hyperthermia, Hypothermia) is sometimes induced in head trauma patients to decrease the patient's basal _____ (respiratory, metabolic) rate.

20. When _____ (hyperthermia, hypothermia) is induced in patients undergoing coronary artery bypass (CAB) surgery, the *measured* PaO_2 and $PaCO_2$ values are _____ (higher, lower) than the actual values when the sample is collected under _____ (hyperthermic, hypothermic) conditions and analyzed at body temperature.

21. For blood gas samples obtained during CAB surgery, temperature corrections to _____ (room temperature, 37°C, patient's core temperature) should be done

during blood gas analysis to accurately measure a patient's ventilatory and oxygenation status.

22. Excessive cooling of the _____ (ulnar, phrenic, median) nerves during CAB surgery may lead to _____ (venous admixture, hypoventilation, blood clot), due to _____ (shunting, paralysis of hemidiaphragms, vasoconstriction).

CHEST INSPECTION

23. Asymmetrical movement of the chest can occur in all of the following conditions *except*:

    A. main-stem intubation.

    B. atelectasis.

    C. consolidation.

    D. tension pneumothorax.

24. Chest expansion is _____ (symmetrical, asymmetrical) when the patient takes in a deep breath and the hands of the examiner move apart in equal distance from midline.

25. A side-to-side technique of _____ (chest percussion, chest auscultation) allows comparison of the quantity of breath sounds between the left and right lungs.

26 to 29. Match the abnormal breath sounds with the related clinical conditions. Use each answer *once*.

BREATH SOUND	CONDITIONS
26. _____ Diminished or absent	A. Pulmonary edema
27. _____ Wheezes	B. Atelectasis
28. _____ Inspiratory crackles	C. Excessive secretions
29. _____ Coarse crackles	D. Airway narrowing

30 to 34. Match the lung segments with the surface projections (landmarks) of these segments. Use each answer *once*.

LUNG SEGMENT	SURFACE PROJECTION
30. _____ Right upper lobe anterior segment	A. Left midaxillary line about 6 in. below armpit
31. _____ Right middle lobe medial segment	B. Left posterior below scapula next to spine
32. _____ Left upper lobe lingula inferior segment	C. Right nipple area (male)
33. _____ Left lower lobe anterior segment	D. Right anterior chest between clavicle and nipple (male)
34. _____ Left lower lobe superior segment	E. Left nipple area (male)

35. Proper identification of the lung segments based on surface projections is useful in all of the following procedures *except*:

    A. charting and reporting.

    B. intubation and extubation.

    C. chest physiotherapy.

    D. chest auscultation.

36. A cuff leak of the endotracheal tube may be detected by placing the stethoscope diaphragm over the _____ (mouth, trachea, lungs). A moderate leak is present if air movement can be heard _____ (at the beginning, toward the end) of a mechanical breath. If the leak is significant, air movement out of the mouth will become evident.

37. Air-filled structures (e.g., trachea, aerated lung parenchyma) do not absorb X-ray, and they are _____ (white-shaded, dark-shaded) (i.e., overexposure) on the chest radiograph.

38. Tissues and bones appear to be _____ (white-shaded, dark-shaded) on the chest radiograph due to high absorption of the X-ray by the tissues and bones.

39. Fluid, blood, and secretions in the lungs absorb a fair amount of X-ray, and they will appear to be _____ (white-shaded, dark-shaded) on the chest radiograph.

FLUID BALANCE AND ANION GAP

40. During positive pressure ventilation, the urine output may be decreased due to:

    A. hyperperfusion of the kidneys.

    B. reduction of antidiuretic hormone (ADH).

    C. increase of atrial natriuretic hormone.

    D. reduction of cardiac output.

41. Monitoring the urine output is important in the management of fluid balance. Oliguria means _____ (excessive, scanty) urine output, and it may indicate _____ (fluid overload, fluid deficiency).

42. Oliguria may occur as a result of:

    A. kidney malfunction.

    B. increased renal perfusion.

    C. increased fluid intake.

    D. increased cardiac output.

43. Normal urine output is _____ (30 to 40, 50 to 60, 70 to 80) mL/hour.

44. Mr. Jones has a urine output of 200 mL in a 24-hour period. This condition suggests fluid overload. _____ (TRUE/FALSE)

45. Oliguria is present when the urine output is less than _____ mL/hour, _____ mL in a 24-hour period, or _____ mL in an 8-hour period.

46. Reduction in cardiac output can be directly attributed to _____ (increased, decreased) venous return secondary to positive pressure ventilation and _____ (increased, decreased) intrathoracic pressure.

47. Positive pressure ventilation also causes a(n) _____ (increase, decrease) in the production of ADH, which _____ (increases, reduces) the urine output.

48. Write in the normal values of the four major electrolytes.

CATION CONCENTRATION	ANION CONCENTRATION
Na$^+$ _____ mEq/L	Cl$^-$ _____ mEq/L
K$^+$ _____ mEq/L	HCO$_3^-$ _____ mEq/L

49. A patient's recent laboratory report reveals the following electrolyte measurements: Na$^+$ = 133 mEq/L; Cl$^-$ = 101 mEq/L; K$^+$ = 3 mEq/L; HCO$_3^-$ = 23 mEq/L. What is the anion gap? Is it within the normal range?

    A. 12 mEq/L, lower than normal

    B. 15 mEq/L, lower than normal

    C. 12 mEq/L, higher than normal

    D. 15 mEq/L, higher than normal

50. Mr. Lawson has the following blood gas and electrolyte results: pH = 7.20; PaCO$_2$ = 35 mm Hg; HCO$_3^-$ = 13 mEq/L; Na$^+$ = 140 mEq/L; Cl$^-$ = 114 mEq/L. Based on his anion gap and acid-base status, his _____ (respiratory, metabolic) _____ (acidosis, alkalosis) is caused by a _____ (gain, loss) of base.

51. Mr. Lawson's metabolic acid-base imbalance (question #50) is present with a(n) _____ (normal, abnormal) anion gap. This is called _____ (hyperchloremia, hypochloremia) metabolic _____ (acidosis, alkalosis) because the loss of base is related to _____ (excessive, inadequate) chloride ions in the plasma.

52. Ms. Johnson, a patient in the kidney dialysis unit, has the following blood gas and electrolyte results: pH = 7.17; PaCO$_2$ = 31 mm Hg; HCO$_3^-$ = 11 mEq/L; Na$^+$ = 136 mEq/L; Cl$^-$ = 99 mEq/L. Based on her anion gap and acid-base status, her _____ (respiratory, metabolic) _____ (acidosis, alkalosis) is caused by a _____ (gain, loss) of fixed acid.

53. Ms. Johnson's condition (question #52) shows metabolic _____ (acidosis, alkalosis) with a(n) _____ (increased, normal, decreased) anion gap. This condition may be produced by the body as seen in _____ (renal failure, alcohol poisoning), or added from an external source as seen in _____ (renal failure, alcohol poisoning).

54. In patients with adequate lung function, respiratory compensation of metabolic acidosis usually takes place in the form of _____ (hyperventilation, hypoventilation).

55. During mechanical ventilation, respiratory alkalosis may occur as a compensatory mechanism for metabolic acidosis. Under this condition, the ventilator frequency should be reduced when hyperventilation is documented by a low $PaCO_2$. _____ (TRUE/FALSE)

56. Severe K^+ depletion can lead to metabolic _____ (acidosis, alkalosis) and compensatory _____ (hyperventilation, hypoventilation).

ARTERIAL BLOOD GASES

57 to 59. Fill in the normal ranges of the blood gas parameters for adults.

MONITORING FUNCTION	NORMAL (P_B 760 MM HG)
57. Gas exchange	$PaCO_2$ _____ to _____ mm Hg
58. Oxygenation	PaO_2 _____ to _____ mm Hg
59. Acid-base	pH _____ to _____

60. Direct measurement of the arterial _____ (pH, PaO_2, $PaCO_2$) via arterial puncture or indwelling catheter is the most accurate method of assessing a patient's ventilatory status.

61. Hypoventilation and respiratory _____ (acidosis, alkalosis) are present when the $PaCO_2$ is _____ (increased, decreased) with a concurrent decrease in pH. This condition may be corrected by _____ (increasing, decreasing) the frequency or tidal volume on the ventilator.

62. Hyperventilation and respiratory _____ (acidosis, alkalosis) are present when the $PaCO_2$ is _____ (increased, decreased) with a concurrent increase in pH. This condition is usually corrected by _____ (increasing, decreasing) the frequency on the ventilator.

63. Tidal volume or frequency control on the ventilator should be used to correct metabolic acid-base abnormalities during mechanical ventilation. _____ (TRUE/FALSE)

64. Patients with depressed central respiratory drive, elevated V_D/V_T, diminished compliance, or respiratory muscle weakness may develop _____ (excessive renal compensation, respiratory muscle fatigue) and _____ (renal failure, ventilatory failure).

65. A(n) _____ (increased, decreased) PaO_2, a(n) _____ (increased, decreased) PaO_2/F_IO_2, a(n) _____ (increased, decreased) $P(A-a)O_2$, or a(n) _____ (increased, decreased) PaO_2/P_AO_2 can be used as an indicator of tissue hypoxia.

66. Ms. Zadori, a 36-year-old asthmatic patient, has an arterial PO_2 of 48 mm Hg while breathing room air. Her oxygenation status can be interpreted as _____ (mild, moderate, severe) hypoxemia.

67. A patient has a P/F ratio (PaO_2/F_IO_2) of 180 mm Hg and PCWP of 12 mm Hg. The chest radiograph shows bilateral infiltrates. These parameters are consistent with a diagnosis of _____ (ALI, ARDS).

68. One of the indicators for acute lung injury (ALI) is a P/F ratio of _____ ($\leq$200 mm Hg, $\leq$300 mm Hg, $\leq$400 mm Hg).

69. A 59-year-old patient has a calculated P(A-a)O$_2$ of 36 mm Hg while breathing room air. The patient's oxygenation status is interpreted as _____ (normal, hypoxemia) since the normal P(A-a)O$_2$ for a 59-year-old should be _____ (more than 36 mm Hg, less than 24 mm Hg).

70. Mr. Protschka, a 55-year-old postoperative patient, has a P(A-a)O$_2$ of 353 mm Hg while breathing 100% oxygen. His estimated intrapulmonary shunt is:

    A. 10%.

    B. 12%.

    C. 14%.

    D. 16%.

71. The normal PaO$_2$/P$_A$O$_2$ ratio should be greater than _____ on an F$_I$O$_2$ of 30% or higher. A PaO$_2$/P$_A$O$_2$ ratio of 60% is indicative of a _____ (hyperoxic, normal oxygenation, hypoxic) state.

72. When hypoxemia is caused by acute hypoventilation, immediate treatment with oxygen should be sufficient. _____ (TRUE/FALSE). Explain.

    _____

    _____

    _____

    _____

73. Hypoxemia caused by ventilation/perfusion (V/Q) mismatch is characterized by a _____ (high, low) PaCO$_2$, and it usually responds _____ (well, poorly) to a moderate level of supplemental oxygen.

74. Hypoxemia caused by intrapulmonary shunting is characterized by a _____ (high, normal or low) PaCO$_2$, and it usually shows _____ (excellent, good, poor) response to moderate-to-high levels of supplemental oxygen.

75. Refractory hypoxemia (hypoxemia that does not respond to oxygen therapy alone) should be treated with oxygen therapy *and*:

    A. mechanical ventilation.

    B. pressure support.

    C. hyperbaric oxygen therapy.

    D. positive end-expiratory pressure.

76. _____ is a mechanism of gas diffusion abnormalities that may lead to hypoxemia.

    A. High oxygen pressure gradient

    B. Increased alveolar surface area

    C. Decreased alveolar surface area

    D. High F$_I$O$_2$

77 to 79. Match the types of gas diffusion defects with the examples. Use each answer only *once*.

DIFFUSION DEFECT	EXAMPLE
77. _____ Low alveolar-arterial oxygen tension gradient	A. Emphysema
78. _____ Increased alveolar-capillary diffusion gradient	B. High altitude
79. _____ Decreased alveolar surface area	C. Pulmonary edema

OXYGEN SATURATION MONITORING

80. In comparison to pulse oximetry oxygen saturation (SpO_2), arterial oxygen saturation (SaO_2) is:

    A. less accurate.

    B. a more invasive measurement.

    C. less expensive to measure.

    D. suitable for adults only.

81. Pulse oximetry may be used to perform all of the following *except*:

    A. intermittent measurement of SpO_2.

    B. continuous monitoring of SpO_2.

    C. measurement of heart rate.

    D. measurement of PaO_2.

82. The heart rate measurement on the oximeter is normally faster than the heart rate obtained by a cardiac monitor. _____ (TRUE/FALSE)

83. SpO_2 above 92% correlates with a PaO_2 above 60 mm Hg. _____ (TRUE/FALSE)

84. SpO_2 measurements are useful in all of the following clinical applications *except*:

    A. assessment of ventilatory status.

    B. weaning from mechanical ventilation.

    C. adjustment of F_IO_2.

    D. reduction of arterial punctures.

85. The recent blood gas report of a patient shows: pH = 7.38, $PaCO_2$ = 46 mm Hg, PaO_2 = 43 mm Hg, SaO_2 = 78%. Since the patient does not show signs of respiratory distress or hypoxia, the therapist should *initially* verify the accuracy of this blood gas report by:

    A. performing another arterial puncture.

    B. measuring the electrolyte level.

    C. measuring the SpO_2.

    D. recommending a stat chest radiograph.

86. The blood gas and pulse oximetry measurements for a postoperative patient are: pH = 7.37, $PaCO_2$ = 47 mm Hg, PaO_2 = 41 mm Hg, SaO_2 = 78%, SpO_2 = 96%. What is the interpretation?

    A. Venous blood gas sample

    B. Moderate hypoxemia

    C. Hypoventilation

    D. Compensated respiratory acidosis

87. SpO_2 and SaO_2 correlate extremely well when the SaO_2 is 95% or greater. _____ (TRUE/FALSE)

88. SpO_2 becomes less accurate as SaO_2 _____ (increases, decreases), and it _____ (overestimates, underestimates) a patient's oxygenation status at _____ (high, low) SaO_2 levels.

89. Sunlight, fluorescent light, nail polish (primarily blue, green, and black), nail coverings, and intravascular dyes may produce a falsely _____ (high, low) SpO_2 reading.

90. Low perfusion and presence of dyshemoglobins may lead to SpO_2 measurements that are _____ (higher, lower) than the actual SaO_2.

91. Mr. King, a patient who was found in a burning house, is reported to have SpO_2 measurements in the upper 90s, while breathing spontaneously on 5 L/min of oxygen via a simple mask. On his transfer from the ambulance to emergency room, the therapist should immediately perform all of the following *except*:

    A. change to a non-rebreathing mask.

    B. change to 15 L/min oxygen.

    C. obtain carboxyhemoglobin measurement.

    D. start aerosol therapy with albuterol and saline.

92. Integrated pulse CO-oximetry is capable of measuring all of the following *except*:

    A. hemoglobin (SpHb).

    B. cardiac index (SpCI).

    C. oxygen content (SpOC).

    D. carboxyhemoglobin (SpCO).

END-TIDAL CARBON DIOXIDE MONITORING

93. End-tidal carbon dioxide monitoring is done to monitor a patient's _____ (circulatory, oxygenation, ventilatory) status.

94. Capnography is a measurement of the partial pressure of _____ (oxygen, carbon monoxide, carbon dioxide) during _____ (the inspiratory phase, the expiratory phase, a complete respiratory cycle).

95. When the sample is collected at the end of inspiration, it is called end-tidal partial pressure of carbon dioxide ($PetCO_2$). _____ (TRUE/FALSE)

96. The major advantage of a mainstream $PetCO_2$ analyzer and the attachments is its _____ (fast response time, light weight, low deadspace volume).

97. The major advantage of a sidestream $PetCO_2$ analyzer and the attachments is its _____ (high deadspace volume, ease of handling, cleanliness).

98. In analyzing a complete capnography waveform, the P_ECO_2 at beginning-exhalation is near _____ (0%, 5%, 15%, 30%) because of the anatomic deadspace volume exiting the airways.

99. The end-tidal PCO_2 ($PetCO_2$) on a complete capnography waveform is the reading taken at the _____ (first, middle, last) part of the waveform at the _____ (beginning, end) of the alveolar plateau.

100. The capnogram can be useful in evaluating or managing all of the following conditions *except*:

    A. esophageal intubation.

    B. endotracheal tube cuff leaks.

    C. hypocapnic management of head trauma.

    D. oxygenation status.

101. The normal gradient between $PaCO_2$ and $PetCO_2$ is about _____ (2, 5, 10) mm Hg in healthy individuals and _____ (2, 5, 10) mm Hg in critically ill patients.

102 to 104. Certain clinical conditions can increase the $P(a\text{-}et)CO_2$ gradient. Match the clinical conditions with the factors affecting the $P(a\text{-}et)CO_2$ gradient.

CLINICAL CONDITION	FACTORS
102. _____ Ventilation	A. During CAB graft surgery
103. _____ Perfusion	B. Increased deadspace ventilation
104. _____ Low temperature	C. Decreased cardiac output

105. A low-cost, disposable, plastic CO_2 (pH) sensitive device may be used as an attachment to the endotracheal tube to assess any occurrence of _____ (hypoventilation, hypoxia, esophageal intubation).

106. Deadspace ventilation (e.g., pulmonary embolism) *or* improvement of ventilation causes a(n) _____ (increase, decrease) of $PetCO_2$.

107. Explain why the ventilator frequency should *not* be decreased when a lower-than-normal $PetCO_2$ is caused by deadspace ventilation.

_____

_____

108. Hypotension and high intrathoracic pressure secondary to mechanical ventilation may cause a(n) _____ (increase, decrease) in $PetCO_2$. Under these conditions, the ventilator frequency _____ (should, should not) be reduced because this $PetCO_2$ change _____ (does, does not) imply that ventilation has improved.

TRANSCUTANEOUS BLOOD GAS MEASUREMENT

109. Transcutaneous blood gas monitoring involves use of a miniature Clark electrode for the _____ (PO_2, PCO_2, pH) measurement and a Severinghaus electrode for the _____ (PO_2, PCO_2, pH) measurement.

110. Transcutaneous blood gas monitoring involves placement of the electrode _____ (over the artery, over the vein, on the skin). A heating element is placed in the silver anode to _____ (increase, decrease) the skin surface temperature to approximately _____ (40°C, 44°C, 48°C) to facilitate the diffusion of gases from the underlying capillaries to the electrode.

111. Transcutaneous blood gas monitoring has been used extensively in neonates and adults. _____ (TRUE/FALSE)

112. In neonates, the $PtcO_2$ closely approximates the PaO_2. In adults, the $PtcO_2$ measures _____ (higher, lower) than the actual PO_2 due to _____.

113. List three conditions that may affect the accuracy of a $PtcO_2$ electrode.

_____

_____

_____

114. $PtcO_2$ is a better predictor of PaO_2 when the PaO_2 is _____ (above, below) 80 mm Hg, and it becomes less accurate when the PaO_2 is _____ (greater, less) than 80 mm Hg.

115. Hypothermia, an increase in skin thickness, and/or a decrease in cardiac output may cause a disproportionate _____ (rise, fall) in the $PtcO_2$ readings.

116. One disadvantage of transcutaneous monitors is the need for site changes every _____ (2, 4, 6) hours to prevent damage of skin caused by the _____ (heating element, tape on the electrode, chemical on the adhesive disc).

117. $PtcCO_2$ monitoring is done to provide continuous _____ (oxygenation, ventilatory) assessment. The $PtcCO_2$ is measured by heating the underlying skin to about _____ (40°C, 44°C, 48°C) to facilitate CO_2 diffusion across the skin to the CO_2 electrode.

118. The $PtcCO_2$ values are usually _____ (higher, lower) than the $PaCO_2$ values. This is due to _____ (increased, decreased) CO_2 production as the underlying tissues are heated.

119. During shock or low perfusion states, the $PtcCO_2$ becomes _____ (higher, lower) than the actual $PaCO_2$ due to _____ (increased, decreased) accumulation of CO_2 in the tissues.

120. Adequate _____ (intracranial pressure, cerebral perfusion pressure) is required to provide blood flow, oxygen, and metabolite to the brain.

121. Under normal conditions, the blood flow to the brain is regulated by the _____ (cerebral vascular resistance, brain's autoregulation mechanism).

122. Following head trauma, the autoregulation mechanism _____ (remains intact, is lost), the cerebral vascular resistance is often greatly _____ (elevated, reduced), and the brain becomes _____ (vulnerable, resistant) to changing blood pressures.

123. The effects of _____ (increased, decreased) cerebral perfusion range from cerebral ischemia to brain death.

124. The critical threshold of cerebral perfusion pressure is between _____ (10 and 20, 30 and 40, 70 and 80, 100 and 120) mm Hg.

125. Select the equation for cerebral perfusion pressure (CPP), where MAP = mean arterial pressure, ICP = intracranial pressure.

    A. CPP = MAP + ICP

    B. CPP = MAP − ICP

    C. CPP − MAP/ICP

    D. CPP = MAP × ICP

126. Based on the relationship of CPP, MAP, and ICP, a higher CPP may be maintained by _____ (raising, lowering) the MAP or by _____ (raising, lowering) the ICP.

127. The normal ICP ranges from _____ to _____ mm Hg. In clinical practice, ICP is usually controlled and maintained at a level of _____ (greater than, less than) 20 mm Hg.

128. In the absence of hemorrhage, the MAP should be managed initially by maintaining an adequate fluid balance and then followed by using a _____ (vasodilator, vasopressor).

129. Systemic _____ (hypertension, hypotension) is associated with poor outcome in patients with severe head injuries.

CHAPTER 10

Hemodynamic Monitoring

INVASIVE HEMODYNAMIC MONITORING

1. Preload is a measurement that reflects the volume of blood _____ (entering, remaining in, leaving) the left or right atrium. It has a pressure unit of cm H_2O or mm Hg.

2. Since the central venous drainage returns to the pulmonary circulation via the _____ (left, right) heart, the central venous pressure (CVP) is known as the _____ (left, right) ventricular _____ (preload, afterload).

3. CVP is measured by a _____ catheter.

4. Afterload is a measurement that reflects the volume of blood _____ (entering, remaining in, leaving) the left or right ventricle. It also has a pressure unit of cm H_2O or mm Hg.

5. Since the pulmonary arteries receive the blood from the _____ (left, right) ventricle, pulmonary artery pressure is called the _____ (left, right) ventricular _____ (preload, afterload).

6. Pulmonary artery pressure is measured by a _____ catheter.

7. The left ventricular preload cannot be measured directly. It is measured by wedging the pulmonary artery with an inflated balloon located at the tip of the pulmonary artery catheter. A small branch of the pulmonary artery is wedged in order to _____ (enhance, stop) the blood flow. The pressure thus obtained reflects the volume status _____ (with, without) the effects of blood flow and vascular resistance in the pulmonary arteries.

8. Measurement of hemodynamic pressures is based on the principle that liquids are _____ (compressible, noncompressible) and that pressures at any given point within a liquid are transmitted _____ (equally, unevenly).

9. When a closed system is filled with liquid, the pressure exerted at one point can be measured accurately at any other point on the same level. _____ (TRUE/FALSE)

10. Complete hemodynamic monitoring is done by using three catheters. Name these three catheters. [Assuming these are not dual-function catheters.]

_____

_____

_____

11. To minimize the effects of gravity, the transducer, catheter, and measurement site should be at the same level. A higher reading may be obtained if the transducer and catheter are located _____ (higher, lower) than the measurement site.

12. Hazards and complications of hemodynamic monitoring include all of the following *except*:

    A. fluid overload.

    B. infection.

    C. dysrhythmia.

    D. bleeding.

13. A PaO_2 measurement of 100 mm Hg in the United States is equal to _____ (1.33, 13.3, 100, 133) pKa in other countries using the Système International (SI) units.

14. Three different catheters are used in hemodynamic monitoring. The arterial catheter is placed in a _____ (pulmonary, systemic) artery. The central venous catheter is placed in the superior vena cava or _____ (right, left) atrium. The pulmonary artery (Swan-Ganz) catheter is placed in a _____ (pulmonary, systemic) artery.

ARTERIAL CATHETER

15. Name four common arteries for placement of an arterial catheter in the systemic circulation.

_____

_____

_____

_____

16. Among the arteries accessible for arterial catheter insertion, the _____ (radial, brachial, femoral) artery is the first choice, because collateral circulation to the hand is also provided by the _____ artery.

17. An arterial catheter can be used to gather all of the following information *except*:

    A. central venous pressure.

    B. systolic pressure.

    C. diastolic pressure.

    D. arterial blood gases.

18. The characteristic dicrotic notch on an arterial pressure waveform is caused by the _____ (opening, closure) of the _____ (aortic, pulmonic, mitral, tricuspid) valve during _____ (contraction, relaxation) of the ventricles.

19. On reviewing a patient's vital signs, the therapist notices that the systemic systolic and diastolic pressures are 100/70 mm Hg. Are they within the normal range? What is the calculated mean arterial pressure?

    A. Yes; 60 mm Hg

    B. Yes; 80 mm Hg

    C. No; 60 mm Hg

    D. No; 80 mm Hg

20. What is the minimal mean arterial pressure required for normal tissue perfusion?

    _____

    _____

21. Given: Pressure = Flow × Resistance. Since arterial pressure is the _____ (sum, difference, product) of blood flow and vascular resistance, an increase of cardiac output *or* vaso-constriction (↑ resistance) would _____ (increase, decrease) the arterial pressure. A decrease of cardiac output *or* vasodilation (↓ resistance) would _____ (increase, decrease) the arterial pressure.

22. Pulse pressure is the difference between arterial systolic and diastolic pressure as shown below.

    A. Pulse pressure = $P_{systolic} + P_{diastolic}$

    B. Pulse pressure = $P_{systolic} - P_{diastolic}$

    C. Pulse pressure = $P_{systolic} \times P_{diastolic}$

    D. Pulse pressure = $P_{systolic} / P_{diastolic}$

23. The normal pulse pressure is _____ (10 to 20, 30 to 40, 40 to 50) mm Hg. Low pulse pressure refers to a ΔP less than _____ mm Hg and high pulse pressure a ΔP greater than _____ mm Hg.

24. A high systolic pressure ($P_{systolic}$) *or* a low diastolic pressure ($P_{diastolic}$) would _____ (increase, decrease) the pulse pressure.

25. A low systolic pressure ($P_{systolic}$) *or* a high diastolic pressure ($P_{diastolic}$) would _____ (increase, decrease) the pulse pressure.

26. Pulse pressure is *least* affected by a patient's changing:

    A. stroke volume.

    B. blood vessel compliance.

    C. heart rate.

    D. spontaneous tidal volume.

27. High pulse pressure may reflect _____ (increased, decreased) stroke volume, _____ (increased, decreased) blood vessel compliance, or _____ (increased, decreased) heart rate.

28. High pulse pressure may be an important factor for _____ (lung, heart) disease, especially in elderly patients.

29. Low pulse pressure may reflect _____ (increased, decreased) stroke volume, _____ (increased, decreased) blood vessel compliance, or _____ (increased, decreased) heart rate.

30 to 34. Match the factors in using arterial catheter with the observed problems. Use each answer only *once*.

FACTORS	PROBLEM
30. _____ Air bubbles in tubing, loose tubing connection	A. Measurement lower than actual
31. _____ Transducer and catheter placed higher than measurement site	B. Backup of blood in the tubing
32. _____ Transducer and catheter placed lower than measurement site	C. Inaccurate reading, signal interference
33. _____ Inadequate pressure applied to the heparin solution bag	D. Dampened pressure signal
34. _____ Blood clot at catheter tip, catheter tip blocked by wall of artery	E. Measurement higher than actual

CENTRAL VENOUS CATHETER

35. The CVP is monitored through a central venous catheter placed either in the _____ (superior, inferior) vena cava near the _____ (left, right) atrium or in the _____ (left, right) atrium.

36. The right atrial pressure can also be measured via the _____ (distal, proximal) port of a properly placed multichannel _____ catheter.

37. CVP measures the filling pressures in the _____ (left, right) heart. Therefore, it is helpful in assessing the fluid status of the _____ (systemic, pulmonary) circulation.

38. CVP may also be used to assess the _____ (left, right) heart function. Because of the catheter position is far from the left heart, it is often late to reflect changes in the _____ (left, right) heart.

39. The central venous catheter can also be used to collect _____ (venous, true mixed venous, arterial) blood samples and administer medications and fluids.

40. The central venous catheter is commonly inserted through the _____ vein or the _____ vein.

41 to 45. In reference to Figure 10-5 of the textbook *Clinical Application of Mechanical Ventilation*, match the waves and downslopes of a central venous (right atrial) pressure tracing with the events during a cardiac contraction.

WAVE OR DOWNSLOPE	EVENT
41. _____ Upstroke *a* wave	A. Closure of the tricuspid valve during systole
42. _____ *c* wave	B. Right ventricular contraction
43. _____ *x* downslope	C. Relaxation of ventricle
44. _____ *v* wave	D. Right atrial contraction
45. _____ *y* downslope	E. Relaxation of right atrium

46. Changes in the hemodynamic status of the heart will cause changes to certain components of the right atrial tracing, particularly the *a* and *v* waves. _____ (TRUE/FALSE)

47. The *a* wave on the right atrial waveform may be _____ (elevated, depressed, absent) when the resistance to *right* ventricular filling is increased as in _____ (mitral, tricuspid) valve stenosis. The *a* wave may be _____ (elevated, depressed, absent) if the atrial activity is absent or extremely weak.

48. Reflux of blood into the right atrium during contraction due to an incompetent tricuspid valve will cause a(n) _____ (elevated, depressed, absent) *v* wave.

49. _____ (Elevation, Depression, Absence) of *a* and *v* waves may be seen in conditions, such as cardiac tamponade, volume overload, or left ventricular failure.

50. The normal range of CVP measured in the superior vena cava is from _____ to _____ mm Hg. When the measurement is taken in the right atrium, the normal value ranges from _____ to _____ mm Hg, slightly _____ (higher, lower) than the reading taken in the vena cava.

51. Since venous return (systemic to pulmonary circulation) is determined by the pressure gradient between the mean arterial pressure and CVP, an increased CVP leads to a _____ (larger, smaller) pressure gradient and a _____ (higher, lower) blood return to the right heart.

52. Since positive pressure ventilation increases the CVP, it leads to a(n) _____ (increased, decreased) venous return and a _____ (higher, lower) cardiac output.

53. The CVP may be decreased in all of the following clinical conditions *except*:

    A. right ventricular failure.

    B. severe blood loss.

    C. fluid depletion.

    D. shock.

54. The CVP may be increased in all of the following clinical conditions *except*:

    A. positive pressure ventilation.

    B. vasodilation.

    C. pulmonary hypertension.

    D. fluid overload.

PULMONARY ARTERY CATHETER

55. The pulmonary artery (Swan-Ganz) catheter is a flow directed, balloon-tipped catheter, and with proper accessories, it can measure all of the following *except*:

    A. cardiac output.

    B. mixed venous oxygen saturation.

    C. arterial oxygen saturation.

    D. pulmonary capillary wedge pressure (PCWP).

56. The pulmonary artery catheter is usually inserted into either the _____ or internal _____ vein. From there it is advanced to the superior vena cava and _____ (left, right) atrium. The balloon is then inflated and the blood flow moves the catheter through the _____ (left, right) ventricle and into the _____ (systemic, pulmonary) artery where it will eventually "wedge" in a smaller branch of the pulmonary artery.

57. After successful placement of the pulmonary artery catheter, the balloon is kept _____ (inflated, deflated) and the catheter stabilized in place. The balloon is _____ (inflated, deflated) only when the PCWP is being taken.

58. List the three components of a typical pulmonary arterial pressure (PAP) waveform.

    _____

    _____

    _____

59. The characteristic dicrotic notch on the PAP waveform reflects _____ (opening, closure) of the pulmonic valve at the end of contraction and prior to the refilling of ventricles.

60. The systolic component of the pulmonary artery pressure waveform may be increased in conditions in which the pulmonary vascular resistance (PVR) or pulmonary blood flow is _____ (increased, decreased).

61. PAP is measured when the pulmonary artery (Swan-Ganz) catheter is inside the pulmonary artery with the balloon _____ (inflated, deflated).

62. The normal systolic PAP is about _____ (5 mm Hg higher than, the same as, 5 mm Hg lower than) the right ventricular systolic pressure.

63. The normal systolic PAP ranges from _____ to _____ mm Hg, and the normal diastolic PAP range is from _____ to _____ mm Hg.

64. Pulmonary hypertension is defined as a systolic PAP _____ (>30, >35) mm Hg or mean PAP _____ (>25, 30) mm Hg *at rest*.

65. Positive end-expiratory pressure (PEEP) can _____ (increase, decrease) the PAP because overdistention of the alveoli compresses the surrounding capillaries and _____ (raises, lowers) the capillary and arterial pressures.

66. Increase of PVR or pulmonary blood flow can also lead to a(n) _____ (increased, decreased) PAP because the pressure measurement is _____ (directly, inversely) related to the resistance and blood flow.

67. Left ventricular failure and mitral valve disease may cause a(n) _____ (increased, decreased) PAP because obstruction or backup of blood flow in the left heart leads to congestion in the pulmonary circulation.

68. The PAP may be decreased in conditions of _____ (hypervolemia, hypovolemia) or use of positive pressure ventilation.

69. When positive pressure ventilation is used on patients who have unstable hemodynamic status, it may lead to a depressed cardiac output, venous return, pulmonary circulating volume, and PAP. _____ (TRUE/FALSE)

70. Positive pressure ventilation (without PEEP) may cause a decrease of PAP due to the resultant _____ (increased, decreased) venous return, _____ (higher, lower) right ventricular output, and _____ (higher, lower) blood volume (pressure) in the pulmonary arteries.

71. In the absence of compensation by increasing the heart rate, a decrease of right and left ventricular stroke volume generally leads to a(n) _____ (increased, decreased) cardiac output.

72. Positive pressure ventilation (without PEEP) may lead to a(n):

_____ (increase, decrease) in intrathoracic pressure.

_____ (increase, decrease) in venous return.

_____ (higher, lower) right ventricular output.

_____ (higher, lower) blood volume (pressure) in the pulmonary artery.

73. The pulmonary artery catheter may also be used to measure the PCWP by slowly _____ (inflating, deflating) the balloon until the wedged pressure waveform is seen. Proper inflation of the balloon usually requires *no more than* _____ (1.5, 3, 5) mL of air. The balloon is _____ (inflated, deflated) as soon as the reading of PCWP is obtained.

74 to 78. In reference to Figure 10-11 of the textbook *Clinical Application of Mechanical Ventilation*, match the waves and downslopes of a PCWP tracing with the events during a cardiac contraction.

WAVE OR DOWNSLOPE	EVENT
74. _____ Upstroke *a* wave	A. Left ventricular contraction
75. _____ *c* wave	B. Closure of the mitral valve during systole
76. _____ *x* downslope	C. Relaxation of left atrium
77. _____ *v* wave	D. Left atrial contraction
78. _____ *y* downslope	E. Relaxation of ventricle

79. A(n) _____ (increase, decrease) of PCWP measurement is often observed in conditions where partial obstruction or excessive blood flow is present in the left heart.

80. The *a* wave of the PCWP waveform may be increased in conditions leading to _____ (higher, lower) resistance to left ventricular filling as in _____ (mitral valve, tricuspid) stenosis.

81. The *v* wave of the PCWP waveform may be _____ (increased, decreased) due to regurgitation (backward flow) of blood from the left ventricle to the left atrium through the incompetent mitral valve.

82. The normal PCWP range is from _____ to _____ mm Hg. A PCWP reading of ≥_____ (6, 12, 18) mm Hg suggests presence of left ventricular dysfunction or left heart failure.

83. The PCWP may be _____ (increased, decreased) during positive pressure ventilation or PEEP due to overdistention of the alveoli or compression of the surrounding capillaries.

84. The PCWP may be _____ (increased, decreased) in left ventricular failure because of backup of blood flow in the left heart and pulmonary circulation.

85. The PCWP measurement may be used to distinguish cardiogenic and noncardiogenic pulmonary edema. In pulmonary edema caused by left ventricular failure, the PCWP is usually _____ (elevated, normal, decreased) along with a near-normal PAP.

86. When pulmonary edema occurs with a(n) _____ (elevated, near-normal, decreased) PCWP, it is probably due to an increase of the capillary permeability as seen in ARDS.

87. A pulmonary artery catheter has been inserted and the presence of artifacts makes identification of the PCWP tracing difficult. The physician asks a therapist to evaluate whether the catheter is properly wedged. The therapist should choose any of the following methods *except*:

    A. postcapillary-mixed venous PO_2 gradient.

    B. postcapillary-mixed venous O_2 saturation gradient.

    C. PAP systolic-PCWP gradient.

    D. PAP diastolic-PCWP gradient.

88. Under normal conditions, the average wedge pressure is about 1 to 4 mm Hg _____ (higher, lower) than the PAP _____ (systolic, diastolic) value.

89. Since a properly wedged catheter does not allow mixing of shunted venous blood with the postcapillary blood, the PO_2 of a blood gas sample from the distal opening of a properly wedged catheter should be at least 19 mm Hg _____ (higher, lower) than that obtained from a systemic artery. The PCO_2 should be at least 11 mm Hg _____ (higher, lower).

90. For the same reason that a properly wedged pulmonary artery catheter does not allow mixing of venous blood, the oxygen saturation value of a properly wedged catheter should be about 20% _____ (higher, lower) than the oxygen saturation recorded with the balloon deflated.

91. Another important value of the pulmonary artery catheter is its ability to _____ (estimate, measure) cardiac output by the thermodilution method.

92. The normal cardiac output for an adult is from _____ to _____ L/min.

93. Cardiac index is used to assess a person's measured cardiac output in reference to the patient's _____ (tidal volume, oxygen consumption, body size) and the normal cardiac index ranges from _____ (1 to 1.5, 2.5 to 3.5, 4 to 8) L/min/m².

SUMMARY OF PRELOADS AND AFTERLOADS

94. Measurements obtained from a systemic arterial catheter reflect the _____ (left, right) ventricular _____ (preload, afterload). For example, the arterial pressure is _____ (increased, decreased) in systemic hypertension or fluid overload.

95. Measurements obtained from a central venous catheter reflect the _____ (left, right) ventricular _____ (preload, afterload). For example, the CVP is _____ (increased, decreased) in systemic hypotension or hypovolemia.

96. Measurements obtained from a pulmonary artery catheter (with the balloon deflated) reflect the _____ (left, right) ventricular _____ (preload, afterload). For example, the pulmonary artery pressure is _____ (increased, decreased) in pulmonary hypertension or blood flow obstruction in the left heart.

97. Measurements obtained from a pulmonary artery catheter (with the balloon inflated) reflect the _____ (left, right) ventricular _____ (preload, afterload). For this reason, the PCWP is _____ (increased, decreased) in left heart blood flow obstruction. The PAP is near-normal in the early stage of left heart dysfunction.

CALCULATED HEMODYNAMIC VALUES

98. The stroke volume (SV) is calculated by which of the following equations? [CO = cardiac output, HR = heart rate, BSA = body surface area]

    A. $SV = CO \times HR$

    B. $SV = CO / HR$

    C. $SV = CO \times BSA$

    D. $SV = CO / BSA$

99. Explain how do changes of contractility, preload, and afterload affect the stroke volume.

    _____

    _____

    _____

100. Oxygen consumption ($\dot{V}O_2$) may be calculated by which of the following equations? [Q_T = total perfusion (cardiac output), $C(a\text{-}v)O_2$ = arterial-mixed venous oxygen content difference, BSA = body surface area]

    A. $\dot{V}O_2 = Q_T \times BSA$

    B. $\dot{V}O_2 = Q_T / BSA$

    C. $\dot{V}O_2 = Q_T \times C(a\text{-}v)O_2$

    D. $\dot{V}O_2 = Q_T / C(a\text{-}v)O_2$

101. The PVR measures the vascular resistance to blood flow in the _____ (systemic, pulmonary) circulation, and it may be elevated in pulmonary _____ (hypertension, hypotension).

102. The systemic vascular resistance (SVR) measures the vascular resistance to blood flow in the _____ (systemic, pulmonary) circulation, and it may be elevated in fluid _____ (overload, depletion).

MIXED VENOUS OXYGEN SATURATION

103. The normal SvO_2 is about _____%. SvO_2 of less than _____% is indicative of hypoxemia or hypoxia.

104 to 106. Some clinical conditions may *decrease* the SvO_2 measurements. Match the conditions with the respective examples. Use *only three* of the answers provided.

CONDITION	EXAMPLE
104. _____ Poor oxygen supply	A. Severe and prolonged hypoxia
105. _____ Excessive oxygen demand	B. Decreased cardiac output
106. _____ Depletion of venous oxygen reserve	C. Cyanide poisoning
	D. Increased metabolic rate
	E. Decreased metabolic rate

107 to 109. Some clinical conditions may *increase* the SvO_2 measurements. Match the conditions with the respective examples. Use *only three* of the answers provided.

CONDITIONS	EXAMPLES
107. _____ Technical problem	A. Sepsis
108. _____ Impaired oxygen utilization	B. Increased physical activity
109. _____ Decrease of oxygen demand	C. Hypothermia
	D. Increased cardiac output
	E. Improperly wedged catheter

LESS INVASIVE HEMODYNAMIC MONITORING

110. _____ (Echocardiograph, Pulse contour analysis, Carbon dioxide elimination) uses the arterial pressure waveform, arterial vascular resistance and patient data to calculate the stroke volume and cardiac output.

111. Lithium dilution and transpulmonary thermodilution are used as reference standards for _____.

NONINVASIVE HEMODYNAMIC MONITORING

112. Transesophageal echocardiography uses the Doppler shift of ultrasound to measure the _____ (blood volume, blood flow velocity).

113. The time velocity integral obtained for the blood flow in the left ventricular outflow tract (e.g., descending aorta) is multiplied by the cross-sectional area and the heart rate to yield the _____ (cardiac output, cardiac index).

114. The transesophageal echocardiography procedure is done by placing a Doppler transducer probe into the _____ (stomach, trachea, esophagus) via the mouth or nose. The distal end of the transducer probe rests at the _____ (upper-, mid-, lower) thoracic level.

115. Carbon dioxide elimination ($\dot{V}CO_2$) can monitor and measure cardiac output based on changes in respiratory CO_2 concentration during a brief period of _____ (tidal breathing, rebreathing, breath holding).

116. The flow, airway pressure, and CO_2 concentration are used to calculate the level of _____ (CO_2 elimination, CO_2 uptake).

117. The original Fick method uses oxygen consumption ($\dot{V}O_2$) and arterial-mixed venous oxygen content difference ($C_{(a-v)}O_2$) to calculate the cardiac output. For the carbon dioxide elimination procedure, a modified Fick method uses _____ instead of $\dot{V}O_2$.

IMPEDANCE CARDIOGRAPHY

118. Impedance cardiography (ICG) is also called _____ (abdominal, thoracic, hemodynamic) electrical bioimpedance.

119. ICG is a(n) _____ (invasive, noninvasive) procedure to measure or trend the _____ (nutritional, hemodynamic) status of a patient.

120. As of 2005, there are two manufacturers of ICG devices using different technologies. _____ (TRUE/FALSE)

121. Impedance means electrical _____ (conductance, resistance).

122. ICG uses _____ (internal, external) electrodes to input a _____ (high, low) frequency, _____ (high, low) amplitude current and measure changes of electrical resistance in the thorax.

123. In a typical ICG set up, _____ (two, four) outer and _____ (two, four) inner electrodes are placed on the patient.

124. The _____ (inner, outer) electrodes transmit a constant, low amplitude electrical current through the thorax.

125. The _____ (inner, outer) electrodes measure the impedance (resistance) to the electrical signal according to the changing blood flow in the aorta.

126. The volume and velocity of blood flow in the ascending aorta changes with each cardiac cycle—increasing volume and velocity during _____ (systole, asystole) and _____ (increasing, decreasing) volume and velocity during asystole.

127. Since the impedance changes reflect the blood flow in the _____ (pulmonary artery, superior and inferior vena cava, ascending aorta), the changes in blood velocity are calculated and reported as values for different hemodynamic parameters.

128. Thermodilution is a(n) _____ (invasive, noninvasive) technique for measuring and calculating the hemodynamic values and it provides _____ (sporadic, continuous) measurements.

129. The accuracy and reliability of the thermodilution technique are not affected by technical factors. _____ (TRUE/FALSE)

130. Among other hemodynamic parameters, ICG can measure and calculate all of the following *except*:

    A. cardiac output.

    B. pulmonary artery pressure.

    C. stroke volume and stroke volume index.

    D. SVR and SVR index.

131. ICG can also provide the values for pulmonary artery pressure, pulmonary artery wedge pressure, pulmonary vascular resistant and index. _____ (TRUE/FALSE)

132. Factors that may affect the accuracy of ICG may include all of the following *except*:

    A. low cardiac output state.

    B. extreme small or large body structure.

    C. presence of pacemaker or arrhythmias.

    D. abnormal cardiac anatomy.

133. Advantages of ICG may include all of the following *except*:

    A. intermittent hemodynamic monitoring.

    B. monitor patient's hemodynamic response to fluids and drugs.

    C. reduced use and risk associated with PA catheterization.

    D. availability outside the hospital.

CHAPTER 11

Ventilator Waveform Analysis

INTRODUCTION

1. Flow-time, pressure-time, and volume-time are three common _____ (modes, waveforms) available on ventilators.

2. Write in the full terms for these abbreviations.

   CMV _____

   FVL _____

   P_{ALV} _____

   PCV _____

   SIMV _____

   TCT _____

   VCV _____

FLOW WAVEFORMS DURING POSITIVE PRESSURE VENTILATION

3. Pressure-volume loop and flow-volume loop use two _____ (modes of ventilation, direct measurements) to create the waveform. In these waveforms, time _____ (is, is not) on the *x*- or *y*-axis.

4. Constant flow waveform (CFW) may also have the _____ (descending ramp, ascending ramp, convex) flow pattern if the rise time to peak flow rate is slowed for patient comfort during volume-controlled ventilation (VCV).

5. During pressure-controlled ventilation (PCV), an exponential decay or concave pattern of the descending ramp flow waveform (DRFW) is dependent on the _____ (lung characteristics, ventilator settings) and patient effort.

6. The ascending ramp waveforms are seldom used or available for PPV because the initial flow rate is _____ (too high, not sufficient) to accommodate synchronized assisted ventilation for most patients.

7. Advantages of using slower flow rates or rise time include _____ (increased, decreased) airflow resistance and improved gas distribution.

EFFECTS OF CONSTANT FLOW DURING VOLUME-CONTROLLED VENTILATION

8. All breaths during volume-controlled ventilation (VCV) are volume- or flow-_____ (triggered, controlled, cycled) and _____ (triggered, controlled, cycled) into expiration.

9. In Figure 11-2, the letter *a* represents the end of _____ (inspiration, expiration) and the beginning of _____ (inspiration, expiration).

10. On the flow-time graphic of Figure 11-2, letter _____ (*b, e*) represents the peak *inspiratory* flow. On the pressure-time graphic, letter _____ (*a, b, c, d*) represents the peak inspiratory pressure.

11. On the flow-time graphic of Figure 11-2, letter _____ (*c, d, e, f*) represents the peak *expiratory* flow. The expiratory flow is _____ (above, below) the baseline or zero flow.

12. Letter *a* on the pressure-time waveform in Figure 11-2 indicates the beginning of _____ (inspiration, expiration).

13. The pressure-time waveform in Figure 11-2 indicates that the breath is _____ (time-triggered, patient-triggered) because there is no negative pressure generated by an inspiratory effort immediately _____ (before, after) point *a*.

14. Refer to the pressure-time waveform of Figure 11-2. The initial rise in pressure (from point *a* to point *b*) is mostly the result of _____ (airflow resistance, total compliance) of the ventilator circuit and endotracheal tube.

15. Refer to the pressure-time waveform of Figure 11-2. The airway opening pressure (P_{AO}) is represented by the pressure difference between points _____ (*a* and *b*, *b* and *c*, *c* and *d*).

16. Refer to the pressure-time waveform of Figure 11-2. Point _____ (*a, b, c, d*) is the peak inspiratory pressure, end of inspiration, and beginning of expiration.

17. In the flow-time graphic (Figure 11-3), the tidal volume can be calculated by:

    A. Constant peak flow × I Time

    B. Constant peak flow / I Time

    C. Constant peak flow + I Time

    D. Constant peak flow − I Time

18. Refer to the flow-time graphic of Figure 11-3. Area *a* represents the _____ (inspiratory, expiratory) or delivered volume. The expiratory volume is represented by area _____ (*a, b*).

19. Under normal conditions, areas *a* and *b* should have similar _____ (pressure, volume, flow).

20. If volume under area *b* is _____ (more than, less than) volume under area *a*, air leak or air trapping may be present.

21. Refer to Figure 11-4. The peak alveolar pressure (P_{ALV}) is also called the _____ (peak inspiratory pressure, plateau pressure). It is measured by stopping the airflow at _____ (end-inspiration, end-expiration) or immediately after the PIP is reached.

22. The peak alveolar pressure or plateau pressure represents the pressure needed to overcome the elastic recoil of the lungs. It is used to calculate the _____ (airflow resistance, lung compliance).

23. The transairway pressure (P_{TA}) is the pressure difference between _____ and _____. Since P_{TA} is the pressure needed to overcome the _____ (airflow resistance of the airways, elastic recoil of the lungs), it is used to calculate the _____ (airflow resistance, lung compliance).

24. (Flow × Resistance) equals _____ (P_{ALV}, P_{TA}, PIP).

25. Controlled mandatory ventilation (CMV) is also called continuous mandatory ventilation or continuous mechanical ventilation. Under this mode, each breath is a _____ (patient-triggered, time-triggered) mandatory breath.

26. A CMV breath _____ (has, does not have) a negative triggering pressure immediately before the beginning of inspiration.

27. Total cycle time (TCT) is the time for each breath from the beginning of _____ to the end of _____.

28. Refer to Figure 11-5. The expiratory time (T_E) time is measured from the beginning of expiration to the _____ (end of expiration, beginning of the next inspiration).

29. Refer to Figure 11-6. The inspiratory flow begins as soon as the negative pressure deflection reaches the preset _____ (terminal flow, sensitivity, plateau pressure) of –2 cm H_2O.

30. The _____ (inspiratory time, expiratory time) would stay the same as long as the tidal volume and average flow are held constant.

31. In the equation $T_I = V_T$/Average Flow, the inspiratory time (T_I) and tidal volume (V_T) are _____ (directly, inversely) related. At a constant average flow, a larger V_T setting would yield a _____ (longer, shorter) T_I. Likewise, a smaller V_T setting would yield a _____ (longer, shorter) T_I.

32. In the equation $T_I = V_T$/Average Flow, the average flow and inspiratory time (T_I) are _____ (directly, inversely) related. At a constant tidal volume setting, a higher flow would yield a _____ (longer, shorter) T_I. Conversely, a lower average flow would yield a _____ (longer, shorter) T_I.

33. Since the total cycle time (TCT) for each breath is the _____ (sum, difference) of inspiratory time (T_I) and expiratory time (T_E), a shorter T_I would yield a longer T_E. A longer T_I would result in a shorter T_E.

34. With PEEP compensation, when the PEEP and sensitivity are set at 10 cm H_2O and –2 cm H_2O, respectively, the mechanical breath would be triggered at a pressure of _____ (–2, 8) cm H_2O.

35. See Table 11-2. Under constant flow ventilation, the volume is the _____ (sum, difference, product) of average flow and inspiratory time.

36. Using constant flow ventilation, a higher flow or a longer inspiratory time provides a _____ (larger, smaller) volume.

37. See Table 11-4. Under constant flow ventilation, the lung-thorax compliance (C_{LT}) or static compliance can be calculated by the equation:

    A. $C_{LT} = V_T/(PIP - PEEP)$

    B. $C_{LT} = V_T/(P_{ALV} - PEEP)$

    C. $C_{LT} = V_T/(P_{ALV} + PEEP)$

    D. $C_{LT} = V_T/PIP$

SPONTANEOUS VENTILATION DURING MECHANICAL VENTILATION

38. In Figure 11-9, point _____ (a, b) shows a time-triggered or controlled breath, whereas point _____ (a, b) shows a patient-triggered or assisted breath.

39. On the pressure-time waveform, patient assist effort is present when the trigger pressure reaches the _____ (tidal volume, sensitivity, pressure limit, peak flow) level. Figure 11-9 shows a sensitivity level of _____ (2, –2) cm H_2O.

40. In Figure 11-10, point d shows the peak _____ (inspiratory, expiratory) _____ (pressure, flow).

41. _____ (PEEP, CPAP, PSV) describes a pressure waveform during spontaneous breathing at airway pressures above 0 cm H_2O.

EFFECTS OF FLOW CIRCUIT AND LUNG CHARACTERISTICS ON PRESSURE-TIME WAVEFORMS

42. As shown in the pressure-time graphics of Figure 11-11, an *increase* in airflow resistance would increase the _____ (PIP, P_{ALV}), while the _____ (PIP, P_{ALV}) remains unchanged.

43. In general, _____ (peak P_{ALV} or plateau pressure, PIP) is not affected by changes in airflow resistance.

44. Peak P_{ALV} is also called _____ (PIP, plateau pressure, PEEP).

45. As shown in Figure 11-12, a decrease in _____ (total compliance, airflow resistance) would increase the PIP *and* peak P_{ALV}.

46. In general, _____ (P_{ALV}, P_{TA}) is not affected by changes in total compliance.

EFFECTS OF DESCENDING RAMP FLOW WAVEFORM DURING VOLUME-CONTROLLED VENTILATION

47. In Figure 11-13, when the flow waveform selection is changed from constant flow to descending flow during time-limited ventilation, the same volume can only be maintained if the *peak flow* of the descending pattern is _____ (increased, decreased, kept the same).

48. In Figure 11-13, when the flow waveform selection is changed from constant flow to descending flow during flow-limited ventilation, the same volume can only be maintained if the *inspiratory time* of the descending pattern is _____ (increased, decreased, kept the same).

49. In Figure 11-13, during time-limited ventilation, the descending flow creates a _____ (higher, lower) *initial* peak flow and _____ (higher, lower) initial flow resistive pressure (P_{TA}) than that created by the constant flow.

50. In Figure 11-13, during flow-limited ventilation, the initial flow-resistive pressure (P_{TA}) is the same for the _____ (sine and accelerating, constant and descending) flow waves.

51. Refer to Figure 11-14. In constant and descending flow ventilation, the rise in alveolar pressure (P_{ALV}) is *directly* related to the _____ (volume delivered, total compliance) and *inversely* related to the _____ (volume delivered, total compliance).

52. Refer to Figure 11-15. During time-limited ventilation at a constant T_I, a reduction in flow would _____ (increase, decrease, not affect) the delivered tidal volume.

53. Refer to Figure 11-16. During descending flow ventilation, a higher end-flow raises the _____ (P_{TA}, mPaw) at end-inspiration.

54. Refer to Figure 11-17. During descending ramp flow waveform (DRFW) ventilation, an increase of inspiratory time leads to an increase of the:

    A. tidal volume.

    B. peak inspiratory pressure.

    C. rise time percent.

    D. A and B only.

55. At end-inspiration during DRFW ventilation, the flow is _____ (60 L/min, zero, −60 L/min) and the PIP at this point is also the peak alveolar or _____ (plateau, mean airway) pressure.

WAVEFORMS DEVELOPED DURING PRESSURE-CONTROLLED VENTILATION

56. In pressure-controlled ventilation, the _____, _____, and _____ are typically set by the respiratory care practitioner.

57. In pressure-controlled ventilation, the flow and delivered V_T are dependent on the:

    A. pressure level.

    B. lung compliance.

    C. airflow resistance.

    D. all of the above.

58. Refer to Figure 11-20. During pressure-controlled ventilation, changes or variations in flow and delivered volume are signs of fluctuating compliance or airflow resistance. _____ (TRUE/FALSE)

59. In _____ (pressure support, volume-controlled, inverse ratio pressure-controlled) ventilation, the patients are usually sedated and paralyzed in order to alleviate patient-ventilator dyssynchrony.

60. Development of auto-PEEP reduces the _____ (PIP, plateau pressure, delivered tidal volume).

PRESSURE SUPPORT AND SPONTANEOUS VENTILATION

61. Under normal operating conditions during PSV, the patient's breathing pattern can affect all of the following *except*:

    A. tidal volume.

    B. flow.

    C. peak inspiratory pressure.

    D. frequency.

62. Refer to Figure 11-22. The first (left) waveform shows that the pressure support breath changes from inspiration to expiration when the _____ (inspiratory, expiratory) flow decreases to 25% of the peak _____ (inspiratory, expiratory) flow.

63. A slower rise time during PSV is _____ (more, less) comfortable to the patient because the preset pressure support level is reached more gradually.

64. PSV is intended for spontaneously breathing patients, and it should not be used in conjunction with synchronized intermittent mandatory ventilation (SIMV). _____ (TRUE/FALSE)

EFFECTS OF LUNG CHARACTERISTICS ON PRESSURE-CONTROLLED VENTILATION WAVEFORMS

65. During pressure-controlled ventilation, an increased airflow resistance or a decreased compliance would reduce the delivered flow and _____ (mean airway pressure, tidal volume, positive end-expiratory pressure).

66. Refer to Figure 11-26. Compare the 1st (normal) waveform to the 2nd waveform. Letter *a* shows a prolonged _____ (inspiratory, expiratory) time, and this observation is likely attributed to an *increase* of _____ (airflow resistance, lung compliance).

67. An increase in airflow resistance will _____ (increase, decrease) the peak inspiratory pressure during *inspiration* and _____ (prolong, shorten) the expiratory time during *expiration*.

68. Compare the 3rd (normal) waveform to the 4th waveform in Figure 11-26. Letter *b* shows a shortened _____ (inspiratory, expiratory) time, and this observation is likely attributed to a *decrease* of _____ (airflow resistance, lung compliance).

69. A decrease in compliance will _____ (increase, decrease) the peak inspiratory pressure during *inspiration* and _____ (prolong, shorten) the expiratory time during *expiration*.

70. Since expiration is normally a passive process, low compliance (high elastance) _____ (enhances, hinders) expiration and results in a shorter expiratory time.

USING WAVEFORMS FOR PATIENT-VENTILATOR SYSTEM ASSESSMENT

71. Tachypnea, agitation, accessory muscle usage, active expiration, muscle fatigue, and respiratory failure are signs of patient-ventilator _____ (synchrony, dyssynchrony).

72. On the flow-time waveform, failure of the expiratory flow to return to baseline is indicative of incomplete _____ (inspiration, expiration), and this condition may lead to _____ (gas leaks, gas trapping).

73. Barotrauma or volutrauma is a complication of mechanical ventilation when the airway pressures or tidal volume are too _____ (high, low).

74. Atelectasis, respiratory muscle weakness, and fatigue are some complications of mechanical ventilation when the airway pressures or tidal volume are too _____ (high, low).

75. A patient is being mechanically ventilated and the sensitivity setting is –4 cm H_2O. Patient-ventilator dyssynchrony is observed. If the sensitivity setting is the cause for this condition, it should be changed to _____ (4, 0, –2, –6) cm H_2O.

76. Prolonged respiratory muscle stress may lead to all of the following signs *except*:

    A. use of accessory respiratory muscles.

    B. active expiration.

    C. paradoxical breathing pattern.

    D. metabolic alkalosis.

77. Refer to Figure 11-28. The solid line of the first (left) pressure-time waveform shows an inadequate _____ (tidal volume, initial flow). This is evident by the fact that the observed abnormality occurs _____ (at the beginning, toward the end) of the inspiratory phase.

78. Refer to Figure 11-28. The solid line of the second (right) pressure-time waveform shows an inadequate _____ (tidal volume, initial flow). This is evident by the fact that the observed abnormality occurs _____ (at the beginning, toward the end) of the inspiratory phase.

79. Refer to Figure 11-29. The solid line of the first (left) pressure-time waveform shows that the patient needs a higher _____ (tidal volume, initial flow) to reach the normal airway pressure tracing (dashed line).

80. Refer to Figure 11-29. The solid line of the second (right) pressure-time waveform shows that the patient needs a higher _____ (tidal volume, initial flow) to reach the normal airway pressure tracing (dashed line).

81. Refer to Figure 11-30. The dashed line (*a*) shows that the patient is _____ (inhaling, exhaling) during the pause time. This maneuver _____ (increases, decreases) the intrathoracic and airway pressures, leading to a rising peak alveolar (plateau) pressure.

82. Refer to Figure 11-30. The dashed line (*b*) shows that the patient is _____ (inhaling, exhaling) during the pause time. This maneuver _____ (increases, decreases) the intrathoracic and airway pressures, leading to a decreasing peak alveolar (plateau) pressure.

83. Refer to Figure 11-31. Compared to the first (normal) flow-time waveform, letters *a*, *b*, and *c* show that the patient's inspiratory flow demand is _____ (greater, less) than that

provided by the ventilator. In this case, the flow or pressure setting on the ventilator should be _____ (increased, decreased).

84. Refer to Figure 11-31. Letters _____ (*a*, *b*, and *c*; *d* and *e*; *f* and *g*) show increased patient-triggering efforts.

85. Refer to Figure 11-31. Letters _____ (*a*, *b*, and *c*; *d* and *e*; *f* and *g*) show incomplete exhalation prior to the onset of the subsequent breaths, possibly due to gas trapping.

USING EXPIRATORY FLOW AND PRESSURE WAVEFORMS AS DIAGNOSTIC TOOLS

86. Refer to Figure 11-32. Compared to the normal **flow-time** waveform (dashed line), the solid line shows a(n) _____ (increased, decreased) peak expiratory flow and a(n) _____ (prolonged, shortened) expiratory time. These changes are likely caused by an increased _____ (total compliance, airflow resistance).

87. Refer to Figure 11-32. Compared to the normal **pressure-time** waveform (dashed line), the solid line shows an increased PIP and a _____ (prolonged, shortened) expiratory time. The change in expiratory time is consistent with a(n) _____ (increased, decreased) airflow resistance.

88. Refer to Figure 11-33. Compared to the normal **flow-time** waveform (dashed line), the solid line shows a(n) _____ (increased, decreased) elastic recoil and a _____ (prolonged, shortened) expiratory time. These changes are likely caused by an increased _____ (compliance, airflow resistance). [Note: ↓ elastic recoil = ↑ compliance.]

89. Refer to Figure 11-33. Compared to the normal **pressure-time** waveform (dashed line), the solid line shows a(n) _____ (increased, decreased) PIP. [Note: During volume-controlled ventilation, *less* driving pressure is needed to deliver the volume when the compliance is *high*.]

90. Refer to Figure 11-34. Compared to the normal **flow-time** waveform (dashed line), the solid line shows a(n) _____ (increased, decreased) peak expiratory flow and a _____ (prolonged, shortened) expiratory time. Lung emptying is _____ (faster, slower) in conditions of low lung-thorax compliance (C_{LT}).

91. Refer to Figure 11-34. Compared to the normal **pressure-time** waveform (dashed line), the solid line shows a(n) _____ (increased, decreased) PIP. [Note: During volume-controlled ventilation, *more* driving pressure is needed to deliver the volume when the compliance is *low*.]

92. In gas trapping, the measured inspiratory and expiratory volumes are usually _____ (consistent, inconsistent) with the tidal volume setting on the ventilator.

93. When gas trapping occurs, the expiratory volume will be _____ (more, less) than the inspiratory volume. In subsequent breaths when the trapped gas comes out, the expiratory volume will be _____ (more, less) than the inspiratory volume.

94. Refer to Figure 11-35. Double arrow *b* shows that the expiratory flow is _____ (increased, decreased) slightly and the expiratory airway pressure is _____ (increased, decreased) slightly. These observations are caused by active _____ (inhalation, exhalation) during the expiratory phase of a mechanical breath.

TROUBLESHOOTING VENTILATOR FUNCTION

95. Failure of the expiratory flow to return to baseline may be a sign of:

    A. gas leak.

    B. airflow restriction.

    C. power failure.

    D. low lung compliance.

96. Refer to the 2nd set of waveforms in Figure 11-36. Letter *a* indicates that the _____ (inspiratory, expiratory) volume is _____ (complete, incomplete) or _____ (more, less) than the inspiratory volume.

97. In gas leak situations during mechanical ventilation, the patient-triggering pressure to reach the sensitivity level may be _____ (increased, decreased).

98. Autotriggering and fast mechanical breaths may develop when a(n) _____ (airflow obstruction, circuit leak) occurs during mechanical ventilation with PEEP. This is because the circuit pressure repeatedly _____ (rises to the PEEP level, drops to the sensitivity setting below the PEEP level).

PRESSURE-VOLUME LOOP (PVL) AND FLOW-VOLUME LOOP (FVL)

99. Refer to Figure 11-38. The difference between P_{ALV} and P_{AO} is _____ (PEEP, P_{TA}, PIP, C_{LT}).

100. Refer to Figure 11-38. On the PVL, a linear increase in P_{ALV} with increasing volume is characteristic of a stable _____ (PIP, PEEP, C_{LT}).

101. Refer to Figure 11-39. On the PVL, a reduction in C_{LT} causes the loop to shift or rotate toward the _____ (pressure, volume) axis.

102. Refer to Figure 11-39. On the PVL, a reduction in C_{LT} will not change the P_{TA} because the gradient between _____ remains the same.

    A. P_{TA} and P_{AO}

    B. P_{AO} and P_{ALV}

    C. PIP and P_{AO}

    D. PIP and P_{ALV}

103. On a pressure-volume curve, an increase in airflow resistance would not change the _____ while the _____ are increased (see Figure 11-40).

    A. P_{ALV}; P_{TA} and PIP

    B. P_{ALV}; P_{TA}, PIP and P_{AO}

    C. P_{TA}; PIP and P_{AO}

    D. P_{TA}; P_{AO}, PIP and P_{ALV}

104. Refer to Figure 11-41. The initial point of inflection (Ipi) occurs when alveoli open in response to an improved compliance during the _____ (inspiratory, expiratory) phase of a mechanical breath.

105. In the presence of Ipi, _____ (PEEP, tidal volume) can be added at or slightly above the Ipi to prevent the alveoli from closing toward _____ (end-inspiration, end-expiration).

106. Overinflation of the alveoli at end-inspiration causes a(n) _____ (increased, decreased) C_{LT} and appearance of an upper inflection point (Ipu).

107. In homogenous lungs (non-ARDS), the strategy to correct the Ipu (point of upper inflection) is to slowly _____ (increase, decrease) the _____ (PEEP, tidal volume) until the Ipu disappears on the PVL.

108. Refer to Figure 11-43. The *expiratory* flow of the flow-volume loop is _____ (above, below) the x horizontal axis.

109. A positive response to bronchodilator therapy would produce a higher _____ (inspiratory flow, expiratory flow) during mechanical ventilation. This is because the _____ (inspiratory flow, expiratory flow) is a ventilator setting.

CHAPTER 12

Management of Mechanical Ventilation

BASIC MANAGEMENT STRATEGIES

1. Ventilator settings such as f, V_T, PSV, and ΔP may be used to directly regulate a patient's _____ (ventilation, oxygenation).

2. The primary strategy to improve ventilation is to _____ (increase, decrease) _____ (one or more, all) of these settings: f, V_T, PSV, ΔP.

3. Improvement in ventilation may _____ (improve, reduce) the patient's oxygenation status.

4. Ventilator settings such as F_IO_2 and positive end-expiratory pressure (PEEP) are used to regulate a patient's _____ (ventilation, oxygenation).

5. In uncomplicated hypoxemia, the primary strategy to improve oxygenation is to _____ (increase, decrease) the _____ (F_IO_2, PEEP).

6. In hypoxemia due to intrapulmonary shunting, the additional strategy to improve oxygenation is to _____ (increase, decrease) the _____ (F_IO_2, PEEP).

7. Improvement in oxygenation may _____ (increase, reduce) the patient's spontaneous breathing efforts and may cause a slight _____ (increase, decrease) in the $PaCO_2$.

STRATEGIES TO IMPROVE VENTILATION

8. Alveolar hypoventilation causes respiratory _____ (acidosis, alkalosis), and it leads to _____ (bradycardia, hypoxemia, metabolic alkalosis) if supplemental oxygen is not provided to the patient.

9. A 45-year-old postoperative patient has the following blood gases: pH = 7.32, $PaCO_2$ = 55 mm Hg, PaO_2 = 58 mm Hg. The ventilatory status of this patient can be interpreted as _____ (hyperventilation, hypoventilation).

10. For COPD patients, the acceptable $PaCO_2$ range is from _____ (30 to 40, 40 to 50, 50 to 60) mm Hg due to _____ (acute, chronic) carbon dioxide retention.

11. Another method to assess the acceptable $PaCO_2$ in COPD patients is to review the patient's $PaCO_2$ obtained at the time of the _____ (current admission to, most recent discharge from) the hospital.

12. A mechanically ventilated patient during postoperative recovery has a recent $PaCO_2$ of 54 mm Hg. The physician wants to reduce the $PaCO_2$ to near 40 mm Hg. The most common method to achieve this is to:

    A. increase the ventilator frequency.

    B. decrease the ventilator tidal volume.

    C. decrease the ventilator frequency.

    D. increase the mechanical deadspace.

13. When the ventilator frequency is over 20/min, the incidence of _____ (pneumothorax, air leak, atelectasis, auto-PEEP) is increased, especially when pressure support ventilation is also used.

14. Minute ventilation = (ventilator V_T × ventilator f) + (spontaneous V_T × spontaneous f). Based on the equation above, the minute ventilation can be increased by all of the following strategies *except*:

    A. increase the ventilator V_T.

    B. increase the ventilator f.

    C. increase the spontaneous V_T.

    D. decrease the spontaneous f.

15. Why is it undesirable to increase the ventilator tidal volume in order to increase the minute ventilation or to reduce the $PaCO_2$?

    _____

    _____

16. A patient who is on the ventilator at a synchronized intermittent mandatory ventilation (SIMV) frequency of 10/min has a $PaCO_2$ of 52 mm Hg. The physician wants to reduce the $PaCO_2$ to 40 mm Hg. Using the equation below, what is the estimated new SIMV rate to achieve this desired $PaCO_2$? [Assume the patient's spontaneous rate, tidal volume, and metabolic rate are stable.]

    New frequency = (frequency × $PaCO_2$)/desired $PaCO_2$

    A. 9/min

    B. 11/min

    C. 13/min

    D. 15/min

17. The patient can help to improve the minute ventilation by _____ (increasing, decreasing) the spontaneous _____ (V_T only, f only, V_T or f).

18. During respiratory stress or when the ventilatory demand is high, a patient usually tries to increase or maintain the minute ventilation by _____ (increasing, decreasing) the spontaneous tidal volume.

19. A breathing pattern consisting of $\uparrow V_T$ and $\downarrow f$ is _____ (more, less) advantageous than one of $\downarrow V_T$ and $\uparrow f$ because a breathing pattern consisting of low tidal volume and high respiratory frequency _____ (increases, decreases) the deadspace-to-tidal-volume ratio and deadspace ventilation.

20. During weaning attempts, for patients who are unable to maintain prolonged spontaneous ventilation or to overcome airway resistance, _____ (PEEP, 100% oxygen, pressure support ventilation) should be tried.

21. The level of pressure support is usually started at _____ (10 to 15, 15 to 20, 20 to 25) cm H_2O, and it is adjusted until the spontaneous tidal volume _____ (increases, decreases) to an acceptable level.

22. Some practitioners prefer to titrate the pressure support level until the spontaneous respiratory frequency is _____ (increased, reduced) to a desirable level. This change in respiratory frequency is usually observed in conjunction with a(n) _____ (increase, decrease) of the spontaneous tidal volume.

23. When pressure support ventilation is used properly, it reduces the work of breathing by increasing the spontaneous _____ (tidal volume, respiratory frequency). As a result of this change, the spontaneous respiratory frequency is often _____ (increased, decreased).

24. Pressure support ventilation increases spontaneous tidal volume, and therefore, the minute ventilation. _____ (TRUE/FALSE)

25. The ventilator tidal volume is usually set according to the patient's _____ (height, gender, body weight) and the range available for adjustments is _____ (very broad, rather narrow).

26. Describe the potential effects of using (A) an excessive ventilator tidal volume, and (B) insufficient ventilator tidal volume.

    (A) _____

    (B) _____

27. The minute ventilation may also be increased by using ventilator circuits with _____ (high, low) compressible volume.

28. High frequency jet ventilation is more effective to improve ventilation in _____ (infants, adults).

29. Why are patients with extremely high airway resistance or low compliance more likely to develop ventilator-related lung injuries?

    _____

    _____

30. Permissive hypercapnia is a strategy used to minimize the occurrence of ventilator-related lung injuries caused by positive pressure ventilation. It may be done by selecting a tidal volume within the range of _____ to _____ mL/kg, compared to the normal setting of about _____ mL/kg. The _____ (pH, $PaCO_2$, PaO_2) levels are allowed to increase beyond normal limits when permissive hypercapnia is used.

31. The incidence of ventilator-induced lung injuries may be reduced by keeping the _____ (peak inspiratory pressure, plateau pressure, positive end-expiratory pressure) below 35 cm H_2O, because this pressure measurement is the best estimate of the average peak alveolar pressure.

32. The small tidal volume used in permissive hypercapnia often causes alveolar _____ (hyperventilation, hypoventilation), CO_2 retention, and respiratory _____ (acidosis, alkalosis).

33. Severe acidosis may cause all of the following conditions *except*:

    A. decreased pulmonary vascular resistance.

    B. central nervous dysfunction.

    C. intracranial hypertension.

    D. neuromuscular weakness.

34. The acidosis associated with permissive hypercapnia may be corrected by all of the following *except*:

    A. renal compensation.

    B. administration of bicarbonate.

    C. administration of tromethamine.

    D. administration of glucocorticoid.

STRATEGIES TO IMPROVE OXYGENATION

35. A recent arterial blood gas report of a patient with chronic bronchitis shows mild hypoxemia. The *initial* method to improve the patient's oxygenation status is to:

    A. increase the F_IO_2.

    B. improve the cardiac output.

    C. start continuous positive airway pressure (CPAP).

    D. use high frequency ventilation.

36. Oxygen therapy corrects uncomplicated hypoxemia because a higher F_IO_2 _____ (increases, decreases) the alveolar-capillary oxygen pressure gradient and enhances the diffusion of _____ (oxygen, carbon dioxide) from the lungs into the pulmonary circulation.

37. Oxygen therapy is very effective in correcting hypoxemia due to _____ (simple V/Q mismatch, intrapulmonary shunting, cardiac arrest).

38. Given: a/A ratio = 0.45. If a PaO_2 of 80 mm Hg is desired, what should be the P_AO_2 and F_IO_2 needed? Use Equation 1 below to calculate the P_AO_2 needed and Equation 2 for the F_IO_2 needed.

    Equation 1: P_AO_2 needed = PaO_2 desired/(a/A ratio)

    Equation 2: F_IO_2 = [(P_AO_2 needed) + 50]/713

    A. P_AO_2 = 118; F_IO_2 = 24%

    B. P_AO_2 = 178; F_IO_2 = 32%

    C. P_AO_2 = 118; F_IO_2 = 37%

    D. P_AO_2 = 178; F_IO_2 = 52%

39. Oxygen therapy is the treatment of choice for hypoxemia due to hypoventilation. _____ (TRUE/FALSE)

40. Hypoventilation is evident when the _____ (pH, $PaCO_2$, PaO_2) is _____ (greater than 7.25, greater than 50 mm Hg, less than 50 mm Hg).

41. A 30-year-old patient who is breathing spontaneously at a frequency of 28/min has blood gases as follows: pH = 7.22, $PaCO_2$ = 58 mm Hg, PaO_2 = 45 mm Hg. The physician wants to improve the patient's blood gases. Which of the following methods is most beneficial for this patient?

    A. Oxygen therapy

    B. Ventilation

    C. Bicarbonate

    D. Oxygen therapy and ventilation

42. Mild hypoxemia that is caused by _____ (shunting, deadspace ventilation, hypoventilation) may be treated by improving the ventilation.

43. Refractory hypoxemia is usually caused by _____ (deadspace ventilation, intrapulmonary shunting), and it _____ (does, does not) respond very well to oxygen therapy alone.

44. Refractory hypoxemia responds _____ (poorly, well) to supplemental oxygen when used with CPAP or PEEP.

45. _____ (CPAP, PEEP) is used for patients with adequate spontaneous ventilation for a sustainable normal $PaCO_2$ and _____ (CPAP, PEEP) is used for patients requiring mechanical ventilation.

46. During oxygen therapy, excessive oxygen should be avoided because of all of the following potential complications *except*:

    A. pulmonary hypotension.

    B. oxygen toxicity.

    C. ciliary impairment.

    D. lung damage.

47. Alveolar ventilation may be improved by _____ (increasing, decreasing) the V_T or respiratory frequency or by _____ (increasing, decreasing) the deadspace ventilation.

48. In _____ (absolute, relative) hypovolemia, the problem is primarily due to volume loss, and the treatment consists of fluid replacement.

49. In _____ (absolute, relative) hypovolemia, the problem is primarily due to loss of venous tone. Fluid replacement should be done with extreme caution because of the potential of fluid _____ (overload, depletion) when the vascular tone returns to normal following fluid replacement.

50. Anemia may lead to hypoxia because the majority (98%) of the oxygen in blood is carried by the _____ (plasma, leukocytes, hemoglobins).

51. Anemic hypoxia is likely when the hemoglobin level is less than _____ (10, 15, 20) g/100 mL of blood.

52. CPAP is useful in the treatment of refractory hypoxemia due to _____ (deadspace ventilation, intrapulmonary shunting).

53. CPAP is only suitable for patients who have adequate _____ (heart, lung) mechanics and can sustain prolonged _____ (cardiac stress, spontaneous breathing).

54. PEEP is similar to CPAP with the exception that PEEP is used in conjunction with _____ (spontaneous breathing, mechanical ventilation).

55. CPAP and PEEP improve oxygenation by increasing a patient's _____ (tidal volume, vital capacity, functional residual capacity) and are therefore very useful in treating hypoxemia due to _____ (deadspace ventilation, intrapulmonary shunting).

56. The table below shows the results obtained from the titration of optimal PEEP using pulse oximetry oxygen saturation (SpO_2) as the indicator. Based on these data, the optimal PEEP is _____ (0, 4, 7, 10) cm H_2O. Explain why.

_____

_____

PEEP (cm H_2O)	SpO_2 (%)
0	81
4	85
7	91
10	89

57. During weaning of a patient who has been using 10 cm H_2O of PEEP and 70% oxygen, the _____ (PEEP, F_IO_2) should be reduced first until it reaches about _____ (5 cm H_2O, 40%).

58. A common application of inverse ratio ventilation (IRV) is for the treatment of patients with _____ (COPD, ARDS, CHF) who are not responding to conventional _____ (oxygen therapy, CPAP, mechanical ventilation).

59. Inverse ratio ventilation improves oxygenation by overcoming the _____ (compliant, noncompliant) lung tissues, correcting the effects of _____ (overdistended, collapsed) alveoli, and _____ (increasing, decreasing) the time available for gas diffusion.

60. Extracorporeal membrane oxygenation (ECMO) is a method used to provide oxygenation of the blood _____ (within, outside) the body of an _____ (adult, infant).

HIGH FREQUENCY OSCILLATORY VENTILATION FOR ADULTS

61. In high frequency oscillatory ventilation (HFOV), the _____ (PaO_2, $PaCO_2$) is controlled by the power (amplitude) and frequency of oscillation.

62. In HFOV, a lower $PaCO_2$ may be achieved by using a _____ (higher, lower) amplitude or a _____ (higher, lower) frequency.

63. A lower amplitude may cause the $PaCO_2$ to _____ (rise, decrease).

64. A higher frequency of oscillation may cause the $PaCO_2$ to _____ (rise, decrease).

65. The mean airway pressure (mPaw) is primarily affected by the _____ (F_IO_2, inspiratory time, power setting, frequency) on a high frequency oscillator.

66. The initial mPaw during HFOV should start at _____ (2, 5, 10, 15) cm H_2O above the mPaw obtained during conventional mechanical ventilation.

67. In patients with severe hypoxia, a _____ (resuscitation, recruitment) strategy may be used during HFOV by applying an mPaw of _____ (20, 40, 60) cm H_2O for 40 to 60 sec by increasing the mPaw in _____ (3 to 5, 7 to 10) cm H_2O increments every 30 min.

68. When _____ (resuscitation, recruitment) strategy is used during HFOV, oxygenation may _____ (improve immediately, worsen in the first 30 min).

69. The lung volume provided by a HFOV may be checked by a _____ (lung function study, blood gas report, chest radiograph).

70. The power setting controls the _____ (frequency, amplitude of oscillation) and thus directly changes the _____ (pH, tidal volume).

71. The initial power setting for adults is set at _____ (1, 4, 8, 10) and rapidly increased to achieve chest _____ (giggle, wiggle).

72. For adults, chest wiggle is defined as visible vibration from _____ (neck, shoulder) to _____ (diaphragm, umbilicus, mid-thigh) area.

73. If the $PaCO_2$ rises (with a pH >7.2), the power setting is increased to achieve a change of amplitude in _____ (1, 5, 10) cm H_2O increments every 30 min until it reaches the highest setting.

74. The initial frequency for adults is set at _____ (5 to 6 Hz, 10 to 12 Hz).

75. If amplitude cannot control the $PaCO_2$, the frequency (Hz) may be _____ (increased, decreased) by _____ (1, 3) Hz increments every 30 min until _____ (3, 9) Hz.

76. A lower frequency (Hz) setting yields a _____ (higher, lower) tidal volume.

77. The initial inspiratory time is set at _____ (25%, 33%, 50%) for an I:E ratio of about _____ (1:2, 1:3, 1:4).

78. The inspiratory time may be increased up to _____ (40%, 50%, 60%) if unable to ventilate the patient adequately.

79. The inspiratory time may be increased by _____ (increasing, decreasing) the amplitude or _____ (increasing, decreasing) the frequency.

80. The F_IO_2 for adult HFOV is *initially* set at _____ (40%, 60%, 80%, 100%).

81. As oxygenation of the patient improves, the _____ (F_IO_2, frequency, power) is weaned to _____ (40%, 6 Hz, 7 Hz).

82. Once the _____ (F_IO_2, frequency, power) is weaned to _____ (40%, 6 Hz, 7 Hz), the mPaw is reduced in 2 to 3 cm H_2O increments every 4 to 6 hours to a _____ (10 to 12, 22 to 24, 30 to 36) cm H_2O range.

83. When weaning is progressing, the patients may be switched from HFOV to _____ (SIMV, PCV, CPAP, BiPAP) where the plateau pressure and mPaw should be kept below _____ (20, 35, 50) cm H_2O and _____ (20, 35, 50), respectively.

ACID-BASE BALANCE

84. Mechanical ventilation may not be indicated in cases where the increase of $PaCO_2$ is a compensatory mechanism for metabolic _____ (acidosis, alkalosis).

85. Respiratory alkalosis is caused by alveolar _____ (hypoventilation, hyperventilation), and it may be the result of acute hypoxia or a compensatory mechanism for metabolic _____ (acidosis, alkalosis).

86. When respiratory alkalosis occurs during weaning from mechanical ventilation, the presence of hypoxia or metabolic acidosis must first be ruled out. Otherwise, reducing the frequency on the ventilator will further induce _____ (hypoventilation, hyperventilation) and increase the work of breathing.

87. If hyperventilation occurs during mechanical ventilation, the ventilator frequency must be reduced *immediately* before the cause of hyperventilation is determined. _____ (TRUE/FALSE)

88. When a patient with COPD is receiving excessive ventilation during mechanical ventilation, acute hyperventilation may cause the patient's arterial blood gases to *resemble*:

    A. partially compensated metabolic acidosis.

    B. compensated metabolic acidosis.

    C. partially compensated respiratory acidosis.

    D. compensated respiratory acidosis.

89. If hypoventilation occurs due to excessive sedatives, the measurement of pulmonary mechanics should _____ (proceed as scheduled, be delayed).

90. Ventilatory (respiratory) interventions _____ (should, should not) be used to compensate or correct primary metabolic problems.

TROUBLESHOOTING OF COMMON VENTILATOR ALARMS AND EVENTS

91. The low pressure alarms are triggered when the circuit pressure _____ (exceeds, drops below) the preset low pressure limit.

92. Factors that trigger the low pressure alarm usually _____ (will, will not) trigger the low volume alarm.

93. Conditions that may trigger the low pressure alarm include all of the following *except*:

    A. loss of circuit or system pressure.

    B. premature termination of inspiratory phase.

    C. obstruction of ventilator circuit.

    D. inappropriate ventilator settings.

94. The low expired volume alarm is triggered when the expired volume _____ (exceeds, drops below) the preset low volume limit.

95. The high pressure alarm is triggered when the circuit pressure reaches or exceeds the preset _____ (high, low) pressure limit.

96. Conditions that may trigger the high pressure alarm include all of the following factors *except*:

    A. disconnection of ventilator circuit.

    B. increase of airflow resistance.

    C. decrease of lung compliance.

    D. decrease of chest wall compliance.

97. List at least three *mechanical* factors that may trigger the high pressure alarm due to an increase of airflow resistance.

    _____

    _____

    _____

98. List at least three *patient* factors that may trigger the high pressure alarm due to an increase of airflow resistance.

    _____

    _____

    _____

99. An acute and severe reduction of lung or chest wall compliance may also trigger the high pressure alarm. List at least three conditions that may cause a reduction of the lung or chest wall compliance.

    _____

    _____

    _____

100. The high respiratory frequency alarm is triggered when the total frequency _____ (exceeds, goes below) the high frequency limit set on the ventilator. This alarm may be triggered in all of the following conditions *except*:

    A. respiratory distress.

    B. excessive sensitivity setting.

    C. high frequency alarm set too low.

    D. circuit disconnect.

101. In the event of frequent triggering of the high frequency alarm, the high frequency alarm may be set higher to disable the alarm. _____ (TRUE/FALSE)

102. Tachypnia during mechanical ventilation may be due to all of the following *except*:

    A. hypoxia.

    B. pain.

    C. excessive inspiratory flow or pressure support.

    D. anxiety.

103. Tachypnia _____ (prolongs, shortens) the expiratory time, increases the mean airway pressure, and alters the ventilation/perfusion relationship.

104. The apnea or low frequency alarm is triggered when the total frequency _____ (goes over, drops below) the low frequency limit set on the ventilator.

105. All of the following conditions may trigger the apnea or low respiratory frequency alarm *except*:

    A. respiratory distress.

    B. circuit disconnection.

    C. sedation.

    D. respiratory muscle fatigue.

106. The high PEEP alarm is triggered when the actual PEEP level _____ (exceeds, drops below) the preset PEEP limit.

107. The low PEEP alarm is triggered when the actual PEEP level _____ (goes over, drops below) the preset low PEEP limit. Failure of the ventilator circuit to hold the PEEP is usually due to _____ (obstruction, leakage) in the circuit or endotracheal (ET) tube cuff.

108. Presence of excessive auto-PEEP may trigger the high PEEP alarm. All of the following conditions may lead to the development of auto-PEEP *except*:

    A. air trapping.

    B. inadequate inspiratory time.

    C. insufficient inspiratory flow.

    D. insufficient expiratory time.

109. Auto-PEEP caused by air trapping may be corrected or minimized by using a:

    A. higher ventilator frequency.

    B. bronchodilator.

    C. lower inspiratory peak flow.

    D. longer inspiratory time.

110. Auto-PEEP is commonly associated with _____ (CPAP, pressure support ventilation), significant airflow _____ (leakage, obstruction), respiratory frequencies of _____ (greater than, less than) 20/min, and _____ (excessive, insufficient) inspiratory flow rates.

111. Auto-PEEP may be reduced by _____ (increasing, decreasing) the tidal volume or mandatory frequency, or _____ (increasing, decreasing) the inspiratory flow rate on the ventilator.

112. Increasing the inspiratory flow rate on the ventilator _____ (increases, decreases) the inspiratory time and _____ (increases, decreases) the expiratory time, allowing more time for exhalation.

113. Auto-PEEP _____ (increases, decreases) the work of breathing because the pressure gradient from the auto-PEEP level to the sensitivity level is _____ (increased, decreased).

114. When setting changes cannot correct auto-PEEP, therapeutic PEEP may be used to reduce the effects of auto-PEEP that is due to air trapping in the _____ (large, small) airways.

CARE OF THE VENTILATOR CIRCUIT

115. The effective (delivered) tidal volume during mechanical ventilation is lower than the set tidal volume, because the ventilator circuit is compliant to pressure and _____ (expands, contracts) during inspiration. As a result, a portion of the set tidal volume _____ (is, is not) delivered to the patient.

116. Given: peak inspiratory pressure = 40 cm H_2O, ventilator circuit compliance = 3 mL/cm H_2O. The volume loss due to the effects of circuit compliance is _____ (13, 80, 120, 200) mL.

117. The volume of circuit expansion under pressure is dependent on the circuit compliance. Circuits with a higher compliance retain _____ (more, less) volume within the circuit and the patient receives _____ (more, the same, less) volume during inspiration.

118. To minimize volume loss due to the effects of circuit compliance, the ventilator circuit should have a _____ (high, low) circuit compliance.

119. A heat and moisture exchanger (HME) may be used as a _____ (permanent, temporary) humidification device for intubated patients.

120. If a metered-dose inhaler is used in conjunction with an HME, the

    A. HME must be placed between the MDI and patient.

    B. HME must be removed.

    C. MDI must be placed between the HME and patient.

    D. MDI must be administered through the nose.

121. The optimal interval for ventilator circuit change is once per _____ (day, week, month) or when it is visibly soiled.

CARE OF THE ARTIFICIAL AIRWAY

122. Patency of the ET tube can be maintained with adequate humidification and prompt removal of retained secretions. _____ (TRUE/FALSE)

123. Since airway resistance is inversely related to the diameter of the tube, _____ (larger, smaller) ET tubes cause an increased work of breathing.

124. According to Poiseuille's Law, when the radius of an airway is reduced by _____ (25%, 50%, 75%), the driving pressure (work of breathing) must be increased 16 times to maintain the same flow rate.

125. Incidence of suction-induced _____ (alkalosis, hypercapnia, hypoxia) may be reduced by using a(n) _____ (open, closed inline) suctioning system and _____ (hyperventilating, preoxygenating) the patient before suction.

126. A closed inline suctioning system should be changed routinely on a daily basis. _____ (TRUE/FALSE)

127. Proper function of the ciliary blanket of the airway is dependent on adequate _____ (oxygen, temperature, humidity).

128. Instilling a saline solution directly into the airway for the purpose of thinning the secretions or stimulating a cough _____ (should, should not) be done routinely.

129. Strategies to decrease ventilator-associated pneumonias include use of proper handwashing technique and all of the following *except*:

A. closed suction systems.

B. continuous feed humidification systems.

C. change of ventilator circuit only when visibly soiled.

D. elevation of head of bed to 5° to 10°.

130. Identification of the microbes that might be responsible for the ventilator-associated pneumonia should be done _____ (once secondary infection becomes obvious, as soon as possible).

131 to 133. There are several potential sources of pathogens that can lead to pneumonia in the mechanically ventilated patient. Match the potential sources with the likely locations. Use each answer only *once*.

POTENTIAL SOURCE	LOCATIONS
131. _____ Patient	A. Manual ventilation bag
132. _____ Health care provider	B. Oropharynx
133. _____ Equipment and supplies	C. Hands

134. The _____ (Gram stain, culture and sensitivity, acid-fast) method of sputum analysis is a technique used to quickly establish the general category of the suspected microbes so that appropriate broad-spectrum _____ (steroids, antibiotics) may be administered without delay.

135. Acid-fast sputum analysis is done to detect infection caused by _____, and silver stain is done to detect presence of _____ pneumonia.

136. _____ (Silver stain, Culture and sensitivity, Acid-fast) is done to identify the microbes in the sputum and select the most suitable type and dosage of antibiotics for the infection.

137. In cases where clinical presentations of an infection point to the most likely _____ (vector, pathogen), empiric antibiotic therapy may be started without a Gram-stain or culture and sensitivity study.

FLUID BALANCE

138. Fluid balance in the body is mainly affected by all of the following factors *except*:

    A. vascular and cellular fluid volume.

    B. pressure gradient of fluids.

    C. electrolyte balance.

    D. heart rate.

139. Water makes up about _____ (20%, 40%, 60%, 80%) of the body weight, with 20% of this volume distributed in the _____ (intracellular, extracellular) compartment and _____% in the _____ (intracellular, extracellular) compartment.

140. When an excessive volume of fluid moves out of the extracellular compartment, an extracellular fluid (ECF) _____ (surplus, deficit) occurs.

141. Mr. Williams, a patient admitted to the medical unit for tachycardia, hypotension, and decreased sensorium, is suspected to have ECF deficit. His problem may be caused by any of the following conditions *except*:

    A. dehydration.

    B. diarrhea.

    C. pulmonary edema.

    D. shifting of fluid into cells and tissues.

142. A(n) _____ (increase, decrease) of urine output is the most common sign of ECF deficit. This becomes evident when the urine output drops below _____ (20 mL/hour, 40 mL/hour, 60 mL/hour).

143. Oliguria or anuria is a _____ (central nervous, cardiovascular, renal) sign of ECF deficit.

144. The central nervous signs of ECF deficit include _____ and coma.

145. List at least three cardiovascular signs of ECF deficit.

_____

_____

_____

146. The treatment of ECF deficit is _____ (potassium, plasma, fluid) replacement with Ringer's lactate solution since its composition is similar to the _____ (blood, ECF, urine).

147. A patient who has severe ECF deficit is being treated with fluid replacement therapy. What are the clinical signs that the treatment is successful?

_____

_____

148. Excessive fluid in the extracellular space is _____ (common, uncommon) in a clinical setting, and it may lead to _____ (loss of sensorium, oliguria, pulmonary edema).

149. The treatment for excessive ECF is to _____ (administer, withhold) fluid or to give a(n) _____ (intravenous fluid, diuretic) such as furosemide.

150. _____ (Lasix, Mannitol) should not be used to treat ECF _____ (excess, deficit) because it can increase plasma volume before diuresis occurs.

151. Since use of diuretics to treat ECF excess will _____ (increase, decrease) the urine output, the volume of urine is therefore a _____ (good, poor) indicator of treatment success. Explain why.

_____

_____

152. A patient who has severe ECF excess is being treated with fluid restriction and diuretics. What are the clinical signs that the treatment is successful?

_____

_____

153. Diuresis often affects the electrolyte composition. For example, Lasix may lead to _____ (hyperkalemia, hypokalemia) and metabolic alkalosis, whereas Diamox may _____ (increase, decrease) the serum bicarbonate level and cause _____ (acidosis, alkalosis).

ELECTROLYTE BALANCE

154. _____ is the major cation in the ECF compartment and it is directly related to the fluid level in the body. Its normal range is from _____ to _____ mEq/L.

155. _____ is the major cation in the *intracellular* fluid compartment and it is not related to the amount of fluid in the body. Its normal range is from _____ to _____ mEq/L.

156. The normal range for chloride ions in the plasma is from _____ to _____ mEq/L.

157. In most cases, once the sodium and potassium concentrations are properly managed and returned to normal, the chloride concentration will be corrected as well without further interventions. _____ (TRUE/FALSE)

158. A patient has the following electrolyte values: Na^+ = 148 mEq/L, Cl^- = 99 mEq/L, HCO_3^- = 22 mEq/L. The anion gap is _____ mEq/L and it is _____ (normal, abnormal).

159. Muscle twitching, loss of reflexes, and increased intracranial pressure are three central nervous signs of _____ (hypernatremia, hyponatremia).

160. Restlessness, weakness, and delirium are three central nervous signs of _____ (hypernatremia, hyponatremia).

161. Fluids that contain no sodium _____ (should, should not) be used to correct fluid deficit. Explain why.

_____

_____

162. Hypernatremia is a(n) _____ (common, uncommon) problem, and it is usually related to water _____ (excess, deficit) as a result of prolonged intravenous fluid administration with sufficient sodium but no dextrose.

163. The normal potassium concentration in plasma is from _____ to _____ mEq/L. It has a _____ (wide, narrow) normal range in the plasma because it is the major cation in the _____ (extracellular, intracellular) fluid.

164. Decreased muscle functions, flattened T wave and depressed ST segment on ECG, and decreased bowel activity are some clinical signs of _____ (hyperkalemia, hypokalemia).

165. Increased neuromuscular conduction, elevated T wave and depressed ST segment on ECG, and increased bowel activity are some clinical signs of _____ (hyperkalemia, hypokalemia).

166. Potassium deficiency may be caused by excessive K^+ loss as seen in all of the following conditions *except*:

A. renal failure.

B. trauma.

C. severe infection.

D. vomiting.

167. When potassium administration is needed, potassium chloride is commonly used because _____ (hyperchloremia, hypochloremia) usually coexists with hypokalemia.

168. Potassium replacement via an intravenous route should be guided by all of the following conditions *except*:

A. urine output should be at least 40–50 mL/hour.

B. KCl should be undiluted.

C. less than 200 mEq of potassium should be given in 24 hours.

D. concentration of potassium should be less than 40 mEq/L.

169. Hyperkalemia is usually due to _____ (hepatic, renal, heart) failure. In acute hyperkalemia, intravenous (IV) calcium chloride or _____ (potassium chloride, calcium gluconate) may aid in antagonizing the cardiac toxicity, provided that the patient is not receiving digitalis therapy.

NUTRITION

170. Poor nutritional intake may indirectly result in all of the following *except*:

    A. depletion of muscle mass in diaphragm.

    B. respiratory muscle fatigue.

    C. hypocapnia.

    D. inability to wean.

171. Interstitial and pulmonary edema may develop in undernutritional status because severe hypoalbuminemia _____ (increases, decreases) the oncotic pressure and causes the fluid to shift into the _____ (cellular, interstitial) space.

172. Excessive nutrition or high caloric intake can cause respiratory distress due to _____ (increased, decreased) oxygen consumption and _____ (increased, decreased) carbon dioxide production.

173. A high-fat diet is more desirable than a high-carbohydrate diet for patients with CO_2 retention because the fat emulsion generates _____ (more, less) calories and _____ (more, less) carbon dioxide production.

174. Based on the Harris-Benedict equation for estimation of a patient's resting energy expenditure (REE) and total energy expenditure (TEE), _____ (more, less) calories are needed for patients under hypermetabolic or hypercatabolic conditions, such as activity, trauma, infection, and burns.

175. Define hypophosphatemia.

    _____

    _____

176. Describe the clinical signs of severe hypophosphatemia.

    _____

    _____

ADJUNCTIVE MANAGEMENT STRATEGIES

177. Use of low tidal volume, prone positioning (PP), and trachea gas insufflation are _____ (routine, adjunctive) management strategies in mechanical ventilation.

178. For patients with normal lung functions, the traditional tidal volumes used during mechanical ventilation range from _____ (5 to 7, 10 to 12, 15 to 18) mL/kg.

179. Low tidal volumes (e.g., 5 to 7 mL/kg) produce _____ (higher, lower) driving pressures than traditional tidal volume (e.g., 10 mL/kg).

180. Higher airway pressures are beneficial and more desirable for patients with acute lung injury (ALI) and ARDS. _____ (TRUE/FALSE)

181. Higher airway pressures increase the incidence of _____.

182. The ideal tidal volume for mechanical ventilation should produce a _____ (peak inspiratory pressure, plateau pressure) of less than 35 cm H_2O because this pressure reading reflects the condition of the lung parenchyma.

183. List three complications of using low tidal volumes (e.g., 5 to 7 mL/kg) in mechanical ventilation.

_____

_____

_____

184. Prone positioning is a way to place the patient in a _____ (face-up, face-down) position in a bed.

185. Prone positioning has been observed to provide all of the following to patients with acute respiratory failure and ARDS with the *exception* of:

    A. higher pulmonary perfusion.

    B. lower airway pressures.

    C. lower oxygen requirement.

    D. lower lung compliance.

186. List at least three goals of prone positioning.

_____

_____

_____

187. Prone positioning improves the _____ (acid-base balance, ventilatory parameters, oxygenation parameters) rapidly. It _____ (does, does not) increase the survival rate of patients with ARDS.

188. The primary indication for prone positioning is ARDS with _____ (increasing, decreasing) oxygen index (OI) while supine and during mechanical ventilation.

189. OI is calculated by:

    A. OI = (mPaw × F_IO_2).

    B. OI = (mPaw × F_IO_2)/PaO_2.

    C. OI = F_IO_2/PaO_2.

    D. OI = PaO_2/F_IO_2.

190. Contraindications for PP include _____ (increased, decreased) intracranial pressure, hemodynamic instability, unstable spinal cord injury, _____ (absence of, history of) abdominal or thoracic surgery, flail chest, and inability to tolerate PP.

191. After one hour of PP, a(n) _____ (increase, decrease) of the OI by 20% or greater from the baseline value suggests a beneficial response.

192. For optimal beneficial effect, pediatric patients should remain in the PP for a period of at least _____ (3, 6, 12) hours.

193. For adult patients, they should remain in the PP for a period of at least _____ (3, 6, 12) hours as tolerated.

194. Which of the following is least likely a complication of prolonged PP?

    A. Accidental extubation

    B. Hemodynamic instability

    C. Tension pneumothorax

    D. Brachial plexopathy

195. Brachial plexopathy is decreased movement or sensation of the _____ (upper, lower) limbs due to impairment of the brachial plexus.

196. Tracheal gas insufflation (TGI) provides a _____ (continuous, phasic, continuous or phasic) flow directly into the ET tube during mechanical ventilation.

197. TGI delivers _____ (1 to 2, 5 to 20) LPM of _____ (oxygen, air, oxygen or air) into the ET tube through a small catheter to the _____ (proximal, distal) end of the ET tube.

198. The gas delivered by TGI exits the ET tube and arrives just _____ (above, below) the carina.

199. When _____ (continuous, phasic) flow is provided by TGI, the gas flow goes into the airway during inspiration and expiration.

200. Drying of secretions, increased tidal volume delivery, development of auto-PEEP, and increased effort to trigger the ventilator are some potential problems of _____ (continuous, phasic) flow via TGI.

201. In phasic TGI, the gas flow goes into the airway during the _____ (inspiratory phase, first half of the expiratory phase, last half of the expiratory phase).

202. _____ (Continuous, Phasic) TGI helps to flush out the ET tube with fresh gas containing _____ (0%, 10%, 20%) carbon dioxide—during expiration, and it fills the ET tube with fresh gas for the next inspiration.

203. During mechanical ventilation of newborns, TGI reduces the instrumental deadspace, improves carbon dioxide clearance, and lowers the ventilation pressure and tidal volume requirements. _____ (TRUE/FALSE)

204. TGI devices have been cleared by the FDA for general use since 2004. _____ (TRUE/FALSE)

CHAPTER 13

Pharmacotherapy for Mechanical Ventilation

DRUGS FOR IMPROVING VENTILATION

1. Airway narrowing is a common complication in patients receiving mechanical ventilation and it can cause varying degrees of respiratory distress. List at least three clinical signs of respiratory distress during mechanical ventilation.

   _____

   _____

   _____

2. During mechanical ventilation, some strategies that are useful in the management of airway narrowing include all of the following *except*:

   A. increasing the high pressure limit.

   B. suctioning the endotracheal tube.

   C. administering bronchodilators.

   D. administering corticosteroids.

3. The sympathetic and parasympathetic nervous fibers are the basic subdivisions of the autonomic nervous system. Stimulation of the sympathetic branch results in _____ (bronchodilation, bronchoconstriction), whereas stimulation of the parasympathetic branch causes _____ (bronchodilation, bronchoconstriction).

4. The neurotransmitter substance released at the *sympathetic* terminal axon is epinephrine (adrenaline), and it elicits a(n) _____ (adrenergic, cholinergic) response.

5. The neurotransmitter substance released at the terminal axon of the *parasympathetic* fiber is acetylcholine (ACh), and it elicits a(n) _____ (adrenergic, cholinergic) response.

6. Bronchodilation can be achieved by eliciting an adrenergic response. This is known as a _____ (sympathomimetic, parasympatholytic) action.

7. Bronchodilation can also be achieved by interfering with (inhibiting) the cholinergic response. This is known as a _____ (sympathomimetic, parasympatholytic) action.

8. Adrenergic bronchodilators (sympathomimetics) are agents that stimulate the adrenergic receptors via the sympathetic nerve fibers of the autonomic nervous system. The receptors thus stimulated include all of the following *except*:

   A. alpha-1 (α-1) and alpha 2 (α-2).

   B. beta-1 (β-1).

   C. beta-2 (β-2).

   D. beta-3 (β-3).

9 to 12. Match the adrenergic receptors with the respective actions. Use each answer only *once*.

RECEPTOR	MAJOR EFFECTS
9. _____ Alpha-1	A. Positive inotropic effect (↑muscular contractility); positive chronotropic effect (↑heart rate)
10. _____ Alpha-2	B. Vasoconstriction, constriction of pupils
11. _____ Beta-1	C. Bronchodilation, peripheral vasodilation, decreased gastrointestinal activity
12. _____ Beta-2	D. Decreased gastrointestinal activity

13. Adrenergic bronchodilators are classified as catecholamines or catecholamine derivatives. Name at least two bronchodilators in each group.

   _____

   _____

   _____

14. Catecholamines have a _____ (rapid, slow) onset and undergo _____ (rapid, slow) degradation. They are _____ (effective, ineffective) when taken enterally.

15. Catecholamine derivatives are considered better bronchodilators than catecholamines. Describe the improved actions of these bronchodilators, and explain what makes the catecholamine derivatives better.

   _____

   _____

16. The adverse effects of adrenergic bronchodilators include all of the following *except*:

   A. tachycardia and palpitations.

   B. sleepiness.

   C. skeletal muscle tremors.

   D. nervousness.

17. Anticholinergic bronchodilators are agents that mainly _____ (enhance, impede) the impulses to the cholinergic receptors of the autonomic nervous system.

18. Atropine is a(n) _____ (cholinergic, anticholinergic) agent that is sometimes used as a secondary bronchodilator. Since it tends to _____ (increase, decrease) the heart rate, it is also used to treat symptomatic _____ (tachycardia, bradycardia).

19. The adverse effects of inhaled atropine aerosol include all of the following *except:*

    A. nervousness.

    B. headache.

    C. bradycardia.

    D. dried secretions.

20. Other anticholinergic agents such as ipratropium bromide (Atrovent) and glycopyrrolate (Robinul, an atropine derivative) are _____ (well, not well) absorbed systemically and, when inhaled, produce _____ (more, fewer) adverse effects than those produced by atropine.

21. During acute episodes of bronchospasm where immediate response is required, ipratropium bromide is the preferred rescue bronchodilator. _____ (TRUE/FALSE)

22. Xanthine bronchodilators (theophylline and its salt form aminophylline) are useful in the management of airway narrowing associated with _____ (infection and trauma, asthma and COPD).

23. For individuals with carbon dioxide retention, xanthines _____ (improve, worsen) ventilation by _____ (heightening, diminishing) carbon dioxide sensitivity in the central nervous system (CNS) and _____ (improving, hindering) diaphragmatic contractility.

24. The three proposed mechanisms of action of theophylline are: _____ (production, inhibition) of phosphodiesterase, acting as an adenosine _____ (agonist, antagonist), and _____ (increase, decrease) of catecholamine release.

25. Xanthines are commonly given via the inhalation route due to their ability to penetrate the mucosal lining of the airways. _____ (TRUE/FALSE)

26. The initial signs of theophylline toxicity include all of the following *except*:

    A. nausea.

    B. vomiting.

    C. constipation.

    D. nervousness.

27. Theophylline toxicity may be avoided by keeping its serum level within _____ (1 to 3 µg/mL, 5 to 15 µg/mL, 20 to 30 µg/mL), the therapeutic range of theophylline.

28. Most of the theophylline is metabolized by the _____ (kidneys, liver, pancreas) and excreted in the urine. Patients at risk for theophylline toxicity are those with heart failure or _____ (renal, liver, pancreatic) disease.

29. Patients with diminished _____ (kidney, liver, pancreas) perfusion due to heart failure or impaired organ function can _____ (increase, reduce) the metabolism and clearance rate of theophylline. These patients are at risk of _____ (theophylline toxicity, bronchoconstriction) due to _____ (inadequate, excessive) serum theophylline level.

30. Patients who smoke _____ (increase, decrease) the level of hepatic enzyme and theophylline clearance. These patients therefore require a _____ (higher, lower) maintenance theophylline dosage to maintain bronchodilation.

31. Corticosteroids are potent _____ (bronchodilators, vitamins, blood components, hormones) that are released from the _____ (kidneys, liver, pancreas, adrenal cortex).

32. Corticosteroids are able to reduce _____ (agitation, inflammation, pulmonary edema), thus making them the drugs of choice in the management of chronic asthma and other similar airway conditions.

33. Corticosteroids have also been used successfully in all of the following conditions *except*:

    A. status asthmaticus.

    B. *Pneumocystis* pneumonia.

    C. drug-induced pneumonitis.

    D. ARDS.

34. Corticosteroids have _____ (strong, moderate, no) bronchodilator effect and _____ (should, should not) be given alone in status asthmaticus.

35. Corticosteroids have an onset time of about _____ (10 to 30 min, 1 to 2 hours, 2 to 24 hours).

36. Corticosteroids return constricted airways to normal by blocking the inflammatory mediators and they should be used when other traditional bronchodilators have failed to relieve bronchospasm. _____ (TRUE/FALSE)

37. List the three general functions of corticosteroids.

    _____

    _____

    _____

38. In long-term use of aerosolized steroids, oral fungal infections (Candidiasis) often occur. They are usually caused by any species of _____ and can be minimized by _____ the mouth after each treatment of aerosolized steroid.

39. Systemic corticosteroids should be used cautiously with patients receiving steroidal-based neuromuscular blocking agents (e.g., vecuronium bromide and pancuronium bromide) because of the potential of _____ (prolonged, shortened) blockade.

DELIVERY OF MDI MEDICATIONS

40. Delivery of MDI medications during mechanical ventilation can be enhanced by all of the following *except*:

    A. synchronization of actuation of MDI with onset of inspiratory flow.

    B. a tidal volume of at least 200 mL.

    C. a longer inspiratory time.

    D. a slower inspiratory flow.

NEUROMUSCULAR BLOCKING AGENTS

41. Neuromuscular blocking agents are used to achieve all of the following goals *except*:

    A. sedating the patient.

    B. relieving laryngeal spasm.

    C. providing muscle relaxation during surgery.

    D. easing management of airway and mechanical ventilation.

42. Other benefits of paralyzing agents include _____ (increased, reduced) chest wall compliance, _____ (increased, reduced) work of breathing, and _____ (increased, reduced) intracranial pressure (ICP).

43. Once a patient is paralyzed with a neuromuscular blocking agent, sedative drugs and opioid analgesics are not necessary because the perception of pain does not exist with appropriate use of neuromuscular blocking drugs. _____ (TRUE/FALSE)

44. At the neuromuscular junction, ACh is the major chemical responsible for the transmission of nerve impulses. It is broken down by _____ stored in the vesicles.

45. When ACh diffuses to the muscle endplate, it produces _____ (repolarization, depolarization) and muscle _____ (relaxation, contraction).

46. A repeating sequence of depolarization and repolarization is required for continued and coordinated muscular movement. Interruption at any point of the sequence causes muscle relaxation or paralysis, depending on the effective dosage. _____ (TRUE/FALSE)

47. One type of neuromuscular blocker binds with the receptor site, producing quick onset and sustaining depolarization. This sustained action _____ (facilitates, inhibits) subsequent neuromuscular transmission and renders further muscle contraction _____ (possible, impossible). Since these agents cause sustained depolarization, they are called _____ (depolarizing, nondepolarizing) agents.

48. There _____ (is no, are several) antidote(s) for depolarizing agents. The length of its neuromuscular blocking action is _____ (completely, partly) dependent on the degree of hydrolysis of succinylcholine by plasma pseudocholinesterase.

49. Another type of neuromuscular blocker does not cause depolarization. It competes with _____ for the receptor sites at the motor endplates, thus blocking the normal action of ACh.

50. Since the nondepolarizing agents compete for the receptor sites, they are also called _____ agents.

51. Nondepolarizing blockers are antagonized by anticholinesterase, and therefore the neuromuscular blocking action is _____ (reversible, irreversible).

52. _____ (Depolarizing, Nondepolarizing) agents have a quick onset but short duration of action, making them the drugs of choice for short procedures such as rapid sequence intubation.

53. _____ (Depolarizing, Nondepolarizing) agents have longer onset times but they are also longer lasting. These drugs are more appropriate for neuromuscular blockade during controlled mechanical ventilation.

54. The degree of neuromuscular transmission and blockade of neuromuscular blocking agents may be influenced by all of the following factors *except*:

    A. organ failure.

    B. drug interaction.

    C. acid-base or electrolyte imbalance.

    D. Rh factor.

55. Patients with altered kidney and liver function have a(n) _____ (increased, decreased) risk of prolonged blockade because of _____ (increased, decreased) drug clearance and _____ (increased, decreased) drug accumulation.

56. Beta blockers, procainamide, quinidine, calcium channel blockers, and nitroglycerine may potentiate the effects of _____ (depolarizing, nondepolarizing) agents.

57. High concentrations of antibiotics may _____ (potentiate, diminish) the effects of competitive agents by decreasing the production and release of _____ (acetylcholine, anticholinesterase). A lower production level of _____ (acetylcholine, anticholinesterase) makes the action of the competitive agents more _____ (intense, subdued).

58. Patients receiving systemic corticosteroids and steroidal-based vecuronium bromide or pancuronium bromide may experience _____ (prolonged, shortened) blockade possibly related to the comparable chemical structure of these two agents.

59. Calcium functions to cause _____ (release, capture) of ACh from the vesicles. An increased level of calcium therefore _____ (enhances, diminishes) muscular contraction.

60. The action of magnesium works in opposition to calcium. An increased level of magnesium therefore _____ (increases, decreases) release of ACh and _____ (enhances, diminishes) muscular contraction.

61. Because of the respective action of calcium and magnesium on ACh, low calcium and high magnesium levels can enhance the effects of _____ (depolarizing, nondepolarizing) agents. Low magnesium levels can magnify the effects of _____ (depolarizing, nondepolarizing) agents.

62. Hypokalemia causes a(n) _____ (increase, decrease) of neuromuscular blockade with nondepolarizing agents and a(n) _____ (increase, decrease) of neuromuscular blockade with depolarizing agents.

63. When neuromuscular blockers are used, acidemia _____ (intensifies, diminishes) neuromuscular blockade, whereas alkalemia _____ (intensifies, diminishes) it.

64. Although many factors alter the action of neuromuscular blocking agents, proper individual dosage can be titrated after the initial dose by monitoring the patient and by meeting the clinical objectives set by the physician. _____ (TRUE/FALSE)

65. The *most* serious adverse effect during use of neuromuscular blocking agents is:

    A. apnea.

    B. loss of coughing mechanism.

    C. muscle atrophy.

    D. psychologic trauma.

66. Use of succinylcholine and atracurium may provoke bronchospasm and hypotension due to release of _____ (ACh, histamine, corticosteroid).

67. List at least three cardiovascular adverse effects of neuromuscular blocking agents.

    _____

    _____

    _____

68. Malignant hyperthermia is a rare _____ (infectious, genetic) condition that can lead to a sudden surge of _____ (heart, skeletal) muscle metabolism when succinylcholine and volatile anesthetics are administered.

69. The increase in skeletal metabolism can _____ (rapidly, slowly) deplete oxygen, generate excessive carbon dioxide, spike body temperature, and cause circulatory collapse.

70. The fastest way to detect malignant hyperthermia is by monitoring with _____ (pulse oximetry, capnography) to detect rapid increase in exhaled _____ (O_2, CO_2) when administering succinylcholine and volatile anesthetics.

71. The preferred treatment for malignant hyperthermia is _____.

72. The peripheral nerve stimulator is used to determine the degree of neuromuscular _____ (paralysis, blockade).

73. The peripheral nerve stimulator consists of two electrodes that are placed along a nerve path where electrical stimuli at 2 Hz are delivered _____ (two, three, four) times in 0.5 sec intervals. This is called a train-of-four stimulus.

74. As the degree of neuromuscular blockade increases, the number of elicited responses (muscle twitches) measured by the peripheral nerve stimulator _____ (increases, decreases).

75. Most recommendations for peripheral nerve stimulator monitoring suggest titration of neuromuscular blocker to _____ (one or two, three or four) twitches in 2 sec. This titration point corresponds with _____ (60 to 70%, 80 to 90%) neuromuscular blockade.

76. The ability to open eyes _____ (slightly, widely), sustain head _____ (nod, lift), and protrude the tongue for more than _____ (2, 5) sec are signs of adequate reversal of neuromuscular blockade.

77. Return of diaphragm function is accessed by acceptable blood gases, maximal inspiratory pressure (MIP) greater than _____ (–15, –25) cm H_2O, and vital capacity greater than _____ (300, 600, 900) mL.

CENTRAL NERVOUS SYSTEM AGENTS

78. Benzodiazepines are used in all of the following conditions *except* in patients who are:

    A. having trouble breathing.

    B. very anxious about the intensive care environment.

    C. undergoing a bronchoscopy procedure.

    D. very combative.

79. Gamma-aminobutyric acid (GABA) receptors are the major _____ (autonomic, central) nervous system inhibitory transmitters. Once the neurons are hyperpolarized by the GABA action, the neurons become _____ (more, less) resistant to repeated depolarization and sedation results.

80. Benzodiazepines _____ (facilitate, inhibit) the action of GABA, thus producing clinical sedation, anxiolysis, anticonvulsant effects, amnesia, slower reaction time, visual accommodation difficulties, and ataxia.

81. Benzodiazepines are usually administered via the _____ (oral, intravenous, intramuscular) route because of unreliable _____ (gastrointestinal, venous) absorption. In addition, pain and _____ (fast, slow) onset of action are associated with _____ (oral, intravenous, intramuscular) administration.

82. Benzodiazepines are metabolized in the _____ (liver, kidneys, pancreas, gall bladder) into active and inactive metabolites that are excreted mainly in the urine.

83. In most clinical settings, the choice of benzodiazepine is often based on _____ (mode of action, speed of onset, duration of action, cost).

84. The physician is concerned about the adverse CNS effects of excessive benzodiazepines on her patient and asks a respiratory therapist to look for any signs of adverse effects. The therapist should look for all of the following signs *except*:

    A. confusion.

    B. combativeness.

    C. drowsiness.

    D. syncope.

85. A patient who has been using benzodiazepines for several weeks is showing the following signs during the weaning attempt: anxiety, tachycardia, diaphoresis, hypertension, and some seizures. The therapist should report to the physician that the patient might be experiencing:

    A. ventilatory failure.

    B. hypoxic brain syndrome.

    C. metabolic acidosis.

    D. withdrawal syndrome of benzodiazepines.

86. Parenteral administration of benzodiazepines may result in a dose-dependent respiratory _____ (stimulation, depression), especially when they are used in addition to _____ (corticosteroids, opioid analgesics, bronchodilators).

87. A therapist is monitoring the hemodynamic status of a patient. The medical record indicates that the patient has been given benzodiazepines during mechanical ventilation. The therapist should expect a(n):

    A. decrease of mean arterial pressure.

    B. increase of stroke volume.

    C. increase of cardiac output.

    D. increase of systemic vascular resistance.

88. Since individual response to benzodiazepines is highly _____ (predictable, variable), monitoring is _____ (not necessary, essential) to ensure correct dosing and cost-effectiveness.

89. Using the Ramsay Scale for Assessment of Sedation, a patient who is cooperative and oriented would have a level/score of _____ (I, II, V, VI), whereas a patient who is asleep with sluggish response to stimulation would have a level/score of _____ (I, II, V, VI).

90. The Ramsay Scale is used to assess a patient's state of _____ (sedation, combativeness, airway reactivity), and it is not suitable for use in _____ (sedated, paralyzed) patients since they cannot perform those commands as required for the Ramsay Scale assessment.

91. To assess the degree of sedation in paralyzed patients, _____ (central nervous, autonomic nervous) signs such as tachycardia, diaphoresis, hypertension, and lacrimation may suggest _____ (excessive, inadequate) sedation or pain control.

92 to 94. Match each benzodiazepine with its respective onset and duration of action. Use each answer only *once*.

DRUG	ONSET/DURATION
92. _____ Diazepam (Valium)	A. Fast onset/Duration is short but may be prolonged if not carefully dosed.
93. _____ Lorazepam (Ativan)	B. Fast onset/Duration is short initially; multiple doses result in prolonged effect.
94. _____ Midazolam (Versed)	C. Intermediate onset/Duration is intermediate.

95 to 99. Severe pain may lead to many different physiologic reactions. Match the reactions with the respective adverse outcomes. Use each answer only *once*.

REACTION INDUCED BY PAIN	SELECTED ADVERSE OUTCOMES
95. _____ Tissue-initiated stress hormone response	A. Delay of bowel and gastric function
96. _____ Activation of autonomic functions	B. Formation of deep vein and pulmonary thrombosis
97. _____ Muscle splinting	C. Increase of blood pressure and heart rate
98. _____ Immobility	D. Breakdown of body tissue and increase of blood clotting
99. _____ Diminished GI function	E. Decrease of ventilatory efficiency and hypoventilation

100. Opioid analgesics produce analgesia by binding to opioid receptors (e.g., mu, kappa, and sigma receptors) in and outside the _____ (autonomic nervous, central nervous) system.

101. Describe the primary CNS effects caused by activation of the mu, kappa, and sigma receptors.

_____

_____

102. Opiates may be further classified depending on whether they are agonists, agonist-antagonists, or antagonists. Opiates that produce a maximal response within cells to which they bind are called _____ (agonists; agonist-antagonists; antagonists), and those that only block opiate receptors are known as _____ (agonists; agonist-antagonists; antagonists).

103. Morphine, meperidine, and fentanyl are examples of _____ (agonists; agonist-antagonists; antagonists).

104. Naloxone (Narcan) is an example of an _____ (agonist; agonist-antagonist; antagonist).

105. Antagonist drugs such as naloxone (Narcan) are primarily used to _____ (intensify, reverse) the effects of opioid analgesics. When these antagonists are used on patients being treated with opioid analgesics, they may _____ (cause, reverse) respiratory depression and lead to the return of _____ (severe pain; spontaneous breathing; severe pain and spontaneous breathing).

106. List the adverse effects of opioid analgesics on the CNS.

_____

_____

107. Myoclonus (twitching or spasm of muscles), convulsions, and chest wall rigidity are the primary adverse effects of opioid analgesics on the muscle group. _____ (TRUE/FALSE)

108. The cardiovascular effects of opioid analgesics include all of the following *except*:

    A. direct vasoconstriction.

    B. histamine release.

    C. bradycardia.

    D. hypotension.

109. One method to prevent hypotension induced by opioid analgesics is to:

    A. use the highest effective dose.

    B. provide a diuretic.

    C. increase the rate of drug administration.

    D. combine low-dose opioid analgesic and sedative.

110. Fast gastric emptying, diarrhea, and vomiting are the primary adverse effects of opioid analgesics on the GI system. _____ (TRUE/FALSE)

111. Other effects related to opioid use include _____ (dilation, contraction) of pupils, altered levels of stress hormones, and uncommon allergic reactions.

112. The precipitation of a withdrawal syndrome on abrupt termination of a drug or after administration of an opioid antagonist is called _____ (tolerance, physical dependence, psychologic dependence).

113. A physician is concerned about the level of pain that his patient may have during mechanical ventilation. He asks you to look for signs of pain. You would look for all of the following clinical signs *except*:

    A. bradycardia.

    B. blood pressure changes.

    C. diaphoresis.

    D. guarding.

114. Explain why barbiturates have limited applications in patients on mechanical ventilation.

    _____

    _____

115. Barbiturates may be preferred in all of the following situations *except*:

    A. seizure disorders.

    B. control of elevated ICP.

    C. management of pain.

    D. head trauma.

116. The normal range for ICP is _____ (1 to 5, 8 to 12, 20 to 30) mm Hg. In clinical practice, the therapeutic goal is to keep the ICP lower than _____ (5, 12, 20) mm Hg.

117. Since an effective hypnotic dose of phenobarbital lasts _____ (1 to 4, 2 to 8, 4 to 12) hours, it is considered a _____ (short-acting, intermediate-acting, long-acting) drug.

118. Barbiturates depress the CNS function via the GABA-mediated hyperpolarization of the neuron, making the neuron _____ (more, less) resistant to depolarization.

119. Barbiturates cause _____ (venoconstriction, venodilation) with peripheral pooling of blood, tachycardia, and depressed myocardial contractility. These events may result in _____ (hypertension, hypotension) especially in elderly patients with _____ (adequate, inadequate) cardiac function.

120. List at least three adverse respiratory effects caused by the use of barbiturates.

    _____

    _____

    _____

121. Barbiturates _____ (increase, decrease) the clearance of drugs that are metabolized by the liver, thus _____ (increasing, decreasing) the effects of those drugs.

122. Barbiturates _____ (do, do not) relieve pain and may sometimes _____ (heighten, depress) the sensation of pain.

OTHER AGENTS USED IN MECHANICAL VENTILATION

123. Other agents commonly used in mechanical ventilation include _____ (nitric oxide, propofol) for sedation and maintenance of anesthesia, _____ (opioid analgesic, haloperidol) for treatment of delirium, _____ (dexmedetomidine, barbiturate) for sedation of mechanically ventilated patients, and _____ (benzodiazepine, nitric oxide) for dilation of pulmonary vessels.

124. Propofol (Diprivan) is an _____ (oral, intravenous, intramuscular) drug administered together with other anesthetics to produce and maintain anesthesia.

125. The mode of action of propofol is believed to be the _____ (enhancement, reduction) of GABA-activated chloride ion channel function.

126. Adverse reactions of propofol include all of the following *except*:

    A. apnea.

    B. tachycardia.

    C. airway constriction.

    D. hypotension.

127. How does propofol contribute to a patient's total caloric intake?

    _____

    _____

128. Since fat emulsion provides an excellent medium for microbial growth, strict aseptic techniques are essential when propofol is used. _____ (TRUE/FALSE)

129. Propofol has _____ (no, moderate, potent) analgesic properties, and additional analgesics are _____ (often, sometimes, seldom) needed for adequate pain control.

130. Propofol _____ (does, does not) promote salivation or vomiting. Its use can be a(n) _____ (advantage, disadvantage) for intubated patients.

131. The infusion rate of propofol should be reduced _____ (rapidly, gradually) to reduce the sudden effects of pain and disorientation.

132. Before haloperidol (Haldol) is used on a mechanically ventilated patient presenting with delirium, a search for the reversible causes of delirium should first be done. Explain why.

    _____

    _____

133. Once other causes are ruled out, haloperidol is used for the control of _____.

134. Haloperidol (Haldol) may be given by:

    A. intravenous route.

    B. intramuscular route.

    C. oral route.

    D. all of the above.

135. Delirium is likely caused by a(n) _____ (increase, decrease) in dopamine release and metabolism. Haloperidol produces a calming effect by _____ (blocking, facilitating) the dopamine receptors in the CNS.

136. What is the primary adverse effect of a blockade of the dopamine receptors?

_____

_____

137. Haloperidol may also prolong the electrocardiographic _____ (ST, QT, QRS) interval that on rare occasions can produce torsades de pointes, a polymorphic form of ventricular _____ (fibrillation, tachycardia).

138. Combined use of benzodiazepine, opioid, and haloperidol may be necessary for control of extremely agitated, delirious patients. _____ (TRUE/FALSE)

139. Dexmedetomidine provides anxiolysis and analgesia _____ (with, without) respiratory depression.

140. The lack of respiratory depression with dexmedetomidine is desirable for the management of mechanically ventilated patients, especially during measurement of weaning mechanics and evaluation of weaning feasibility. _____ (TRUE/FALSE)

141. Indications for dexmedetomidine include all of the following *except*:

   A. control of intracranial pressure.

   B. pre-, during, and post-extubation.

   C. prior to and during cardiac or vascular surgeries.

   D. intranasally for children undergoing MRI and CT procedures.

142. Dexmedetomidine is an α_2 adrenoreceptor _____ (agonist, antagonist) which provides sedation and anxiolysis via receptors within the locus ceruleus (group of neurons in the pons), and analgesia via receptors in the spinal cord.

143. Adverse reactions of dexmedetomidine include _____ (hypertension, hypotension, _____ (tachycardia, bradycardia) and sinus _____ (tachycardia, arrest).

144. Mild _____ (hypertension, hypotension) due to dexmedetomidine may be managed by increasing the rate of intravenous fluid, elevating the lower extremities, and using vasopressors.

145. Inhaled NO therapy is currently being evaluated for its potential application in all of the following conditions *except*:

   A. congenital heart disease.

   B. persistent pulmonary hypertension of the newborn.

   C. pleural effusion.

   D. respiratory distress syndrome.

146. Inhaled NO produces local _____ (vasodilation, vasoconstriction) of vascular smooth muscles in the lung, and it reduces pulmonary vascular resistance, corrects V/Q mismatch, and improves oxygenation.

147. Why are the by-products of inhaled NO harmful to the lungs?

_____

_____

148. Inhaled NO is inactivated by combining with hemoglobin to form _____, a form of hemoglobin in blood that is incapable of transporting oxygen.

149. The appearance of a patient with 10 to 20% of methemoglobin is usually _____ (symptomatic, asymptomatic) but _____ (may, may not) have central cyanosis of trunk and limbs.

150. CNS depression (headache, dizziness, fatigue, lethargy, syncope) may be observed when the methemoglobin level is between _____ (0% and 5%; 20% and 45%, 50% and 70%).

151. For patient benefit and safety, the delivery system for inhaled NO therapy should be able to deliver a _____ (constant, fluctuating) percent of NO and to provide _____ (continuous, intermittent) monitoring of NO, NO_2, and O_2.

CHAPTER 14

Procedures Related to Mechanical Ventilation

CHEST TUBE AND DRAINAGE SYSTEM

1. A chest tube is also called a _____ that is connected to the _____ and drainage system for removal of air or fluid.

2. Common indications for placement of a chest tube include all of the following conditions *except*:

   A. tension pneumothorax.

   B. pneumonia.

   C. hemothorax.

   D. pleural effusion.

3. Infection over the insertion site and conditions that may lead to severe bleeding are _____ (absolute, relative) contraindications to chest tube placement.

4. Hemorrhage at the insertion site, hematoma, and laceration of lung parenchyma or intraabdominal organs are some complications _____ (during, three days following) chest tube placement.

5. Infection can be one of the _____ (early, late) complications of chest tube placement.

6. Trocar is a _____ (sharp, blunt) instrument for incision into the chest cavity.

7. The suggested chest tube size for large adults ranges from 36 to 40 _____ (cm, mm, Fr).

8. The suggested chest tube size for small adults or teens ranges from _____ (18 to 20, 22 to 26, 28 to 32) Fr.

9. The suggested chest tube size for _____ (small adults, children, neonates) is about 18 Fr.

10. Since clotting of the chest tube with blood or pleural fluid is less likely in pneumothoraces, chest tube size from _____ (10 to 14, 16 to 20) Fr may be adequate for adults.

11. Describe the recommended location of chest tube placement for treatment of pneumothorax.

   _____

   _____

12. Describe the recommended location of chest tube placement for drainage of pleural fluid.

   _____

   _____

13. During chest tube placement, the point of entry is directly _____ (over, below) the body of the rib because arteries, veins, and intercostal nerves all lie _____ (above, below) each rib.

14. _____ (Operative, Trocar) tube thoracostomy is a technique of test tube placement by dissection into the pleura, digital inspection of the pleural space, and insertion guided with the finger and hemostat.

15. Compared to operative tube thoracostomy, trocar tube thoracostomy requires a _____ (larger, smaller) incision, and it carries a _____ (higher, lower) risk of puncturing the lung.

16. Kinking of the chest tube will lower the suction level, hinder lung reexpansion, and cause the fluid to enter the pleural space. _____ (TRUE/FALSE)

17. A three-chamber drainage system used for evacuation of pleural fluid _____ (does, does not) require a vacuum source for proper operation.

18. When a one-chamber system is used to evacuate pleural fluid, accumulation of pleural fluid in the system will _____ (enhance, hinder) spontaneous breathing.

19. When a two-chamber system is used to evacuate pleural fluid, accumulation of pleural fluid in the system _____ (will, will not) affect the spontaneous breathing effort.

20. In a three-chamber drainage system, chamber 1 (proximal to the patient) is called the _____ (collection, water seal, suction) chamber.

21. The amount of suction in the three-chamber chest tube drainage system is regulated by the:

   A. vacuum setting.

   B. fluid level in chamber 1 (proximal to the patient).

   C. fluid level in chamber 2.

   D. fluid level in chamber 3 (distal to the patient).

22. Chamber 2 is the _____ (collection, water seal, suction) chamber in a three-chamber chest tube drainage system.

23. If a suction level of -10 cm H_2O is desired, sterile water should be added to the chamber _____ (proximal, distal) to the patient until it reaches a height of _____ cm H_2O.

24. The water level in chamber 3 (distal to the patient) regulates the amount of _____ (drainage, suction) in the three-chamber system.

25. A suction level of _____ (−5 to −10, −10 to −20, −20 to −30) cm H_2O is recommended for the chest tube drainage system.

26. The setting of wall vacuum and the amount of bubbling reflects the level of suction applied to the pleural space. _____ (TRUE/FALSE)

27. Too much bubbling in chamber 3 (distal to the patient) of a three-chamber chest tube drainage system means the:

    A. vacuum level is set too high.

    B. suction to the pleural space is too much.

    C. collection chamber is full.

    D. drainage system has a leak.

28. The level of suction applied to the pleural space is determined by the submersion depth of the venting tube in the _____ (collection, water seal, suction) chamber.

29. Evaporation losses of fluid in the suction chamber will _____ (increase, decrease) the suction level to the pleural space.

30. When the water level in the middle (water seal) chamber fluctuates with respiration, it means that the tube and drainage system:

    A. are working properly.

    B. have a leak.

    C. are occluded.

    D. have too much suction.

31. A large amount of bubbling in the water seal chamber 2 (middle chamber) suggests:

    A. an air leak in the drainage system.

    B. the presence of air in the pleural space.

    C. that the vacuum is too high.

    D. A and B only.

32. Overfilling of water in chamber 3 (distal to patient) will _____ (increase, decrease) the suction level to the pleural space, whereas underfilling will _____ (increase, decrease) the suction level.

33. The chest tube can be removed when the drainage has stopped or slowed to less than _____ (100 mL, 300 mL, 500 mL) over 24 hours.

34. The chest tube can be removed when the pneumothorax has resolved and there is no further air leak. Air leak (i.e., bubbling) in the _____ (collection, water seal, suction) chamber may be tested by asking the patient to perform a Valsalva maneuver or a forceful cough.

35. During transport of a patient with a chest tube, the drainage system must be kept _____ (higher, lower) than the patient's chest, and the chest tube must not be clamped or occluded.

36. During patient transport, prolonged clamping of the chest tube is permissible if a chest tube drainage system is not readily available. _____ (TRUE/FALSE)

ASSISTING IN FIBEROPTIC BRONCHOSCOPY

37. A fiberoptic bronchoscope is an instrument that uses _____ (plastic, glass, silicone) fibers to transmit images of the airway.

38. Fiberoptic bronchoscopy facilitates or provides all of the following *diagnostic* uses with the *exception* of:

    A. evaluation and diagnosis of hemoptysis.

    B. collection of biopsy or cytology samples.

    C. staging of lung cancer.

    D. insertion of difficult airway.

39. Evaluation of vocal cords paralysis is an example of _____ (diagnostic, therapeutic) bronchoscopy.

40. The indications for *therapeutic* bronchoscopy include all of the following *except*:

    A. removal of secretions not mobilized by conventional techniques.

    B. administration of bronchodilator.

    C. removal of foreign bodies in medium airway.

    D. intubation of difficult airway.

41. The _____ (handle, videoscope, channel outlet) of a bronchoscope is used for installation of saline or topical anesthetics, suction, and for passage of biopsy forceps.

42. _____ (Diazepam, Atropine sulfate, Lidocaine, Morphine sulfate) is given to the patient _____ (intravenously, via aerosol) 30 min before the bronchoscopy procedure to reduce irritation of the mucosal membrane.

43. The recommended dosage for lidocaine is _____ (1 to 3 mL, 5 to 10 mL) of a _____ (1 to 4%, 5 to 10%) solution.

44. _____ (Diazepam, Atropine sulfate, Lidocaine, Morphine sulfate) is given to reduce vagal response, oral secretions, and bronchospasm.

45. To provide pain relief and suppress coughing during bronchoscopy, _____ may be used.

46. Diazepam or a suitable benzodiazepine is given intravenously in bolus to provide _____ (pain relief, sedation) during bronchoscopy.

47. The insertion tube of a bronchoscope may be inserted via the nares, mouth (with bit block), endotracheal tube, or tracheostomy tube. _____ (TRUE/FALSE)

48. The insertion tube of a bronchoscope should not be inserted via the tracheostomy tube. _____ (TRUE/FALSE)

49. The amount of oxygen provided to a patient undergoing bronchoscopy may be titrated using a(n) _____ (oxygen analyzer, pulse oximeter, oxygen blender).

50. When bronchoscopy is done on patients receiving mechanical ventilation, minor air leak may be compensated by increasing the _____ (frequency, PEEP, tidal volume), and the pressure limit may need to be _____ (increased, decreased) to compensate for a larger tidal volume and insertion tube in the endotracheal tube.

51. During collection of secretions with a bronchoscope, pulmonary lavage with a _____ (sterile water, saline) solution is sometimes necessary for thick secretions.

52. Forceps biopsy is done to collect _____ (secretion, tissue) specimens from the airway or lung parenchyma.

53. _____ (Transbronchial needle aspiration biopsy, Transbronchial lung biopsy, Forceps biopsy) is done to collect tissue specimens using a forced exhalation maneuver.

54. Transbronchial needle aspiration biopsy is done where the lesion is located _____ (next to, beyond) the bronchial wall and there _____ (is, is no) lesion in the bronchial lumen.

55. Bronchial brushing is done to collect _____ (secretions, tissue or loosened cell specimens) via a bronchoscope.

56. Infection is rarely a complication of bronchoscopy. _____ (TRUE/FALSE)

57. Bleeding during bronchoscopy may be stopped by all of the following techniques *except*:

    A. using heat-induced coagulation.

    B. wedging the bleeding site with the distal end of the bronchoscope.

    C. plugging the airway where bleeding occurs.

    D. using a vasopressor.

58. Worsening cyanosis in spite of high oxygen concentration, diaphoresis, tachypnea, tachycardia, and thready pulse are some signs of tension pneumothorax. _____ (TRUE/FALSE)

59. _____ (Tension pneumothorax, Hypoxemia and arrhythmias) are the most common complications during and after bronchoscopy.

60. Following bronchoscopy, food and drinks are withheld from the patient until the _____ (normal SpO$_2$, normal blood gases, gag reflex) has returned.

61. Following bronchoscopy, the portions of the bronchoscope that have come in contact with the mucosal membrane must be _____ (disinfected, sterilized).

TRANSPORT OF MECHANICALLY VENTILATED PATIENTS

62. The available resources during transport of mechanically ventilated patients are typically _____ (more than, same as, less than) that available in the intensive care unit.

63. The most common indication for *intrahospital* transport of mechanically ventilated patients is to acquire _____ (diagnostic procedures, tertiary medical care or procedures).

64. The usual indication for *interhospital* transport of mechanically ventilated patients is to acquire _____ (diagnostic procedures, tertiary medical care or procedures).

65. All of the following may be contraindications for an urgent transport of mechanically ventilated patients *except*:

   A. inability to provide adequate oxygenation and ventilation.

   B. inability to maintain acceptable hemodynamic status.

   C. inability to provide adequate airway control or cardiopulmonary monitoring.

   D. insufficient nursing and respiratory care staff in the intensive care unit (ICU).

66. A mechanically ventilated patient may undergo transport as quickly as possible when the hemodynamic status is deteriorating. _____ (TRUE/FALSE)

67 to 70. Match the type of equipment and supplies for the transport of mechanically ventilated patients in Column I with the respective examples in Column II. Use *only* four answers in Column II.

COLUMN I: TYPE OF EQUIPMENT	COLUMN II: EXAMPLES AND SUPPLIES
67. _____ Standard precaution	A. Oxygen cylinders (full and with wrench)
68. _____ Patient assessment and monitoring	B. Intubation supplies (laryngoscope handles and blades, fresh batteries, endotracheal tubes, etc.)
69. _____ Airway management	C. Epinephrine
70. _____ Oxygenation supplies	D. Stethoscopes
	E. Gloves (sterile and clean)

71. For interhospital transport, the selection of the mode of transportation is mainly based on the:

   A. number of transport personnel.

   B. distance between hospitals.

   C. cost of transport.

   D. age of the patient being transported.

72. Which of the following modes of transportation is least likely being used for transport of mechanically ventilated patients in the United States? _____ (Ground ambulance, Boat, Helicopter, Propeller-drive aircraft, Jet).

73. A transport ventilator requires a piped-in gas source and electrical connection for normal operation. _____ (TRUE/FALSE)

74. Patient transport by _____ (ground ambulance, helicopter, propeller-driven aircraft, jet) is limited by road and traffic conditions.

75. _____ (Ground ambulance, Helicopter, Propeller-driven aircraft, Jet) is the choice for patient transport to another facility 300 miles away.

76. Low P_IO_2 and relative humidity are two inherited problems at high altitude in _____ (pressurized, nonpressurized) aircrafts.

77. For intrahospital transport of patients who require ventilatory support for a short time (e.g., less than 30 min), manual ventilation with a resuscitation bag and oxygen may be sufficient. _____ (TRUE/FALSE)

78. Manual ventilation may lead to inadvertent _____ (hypoventilation, hyperventilation) and _____ (regular, irregular) tidal volume and frequency.

79. There are three brands of transport ventilators available in the United States. _____ (TRUE/FALSE)

80. Most transport ventilators have features such as PEEP, pressure support ventilation, volume- and pressure-controlled ventilation, and inverse ratio ventilation. _____ (TRUE/FALSE)

81. For ventilators that operate with only the pressure-controlled mode, the _____ (peak inspiratory pressure, expired volume) must be monitored closely since decreasing compliance or increasing airflow resistance can lead to decreasing _____ (plateau pressure, tidal volume).

82. The patient using a jet for intercontinental transport is _____ (usually, rarely) in critical condition due to the time required for planning and the long flight time.

83. A written physician order _____ (is, is not) required prior to transporting a mechanically ventilated patient.

84. During transport, the patient is monitored _____ (at the beginning of transport, toward the end of transport, throughout the entire period) to ensure stable hemodynamic status and adequate oxygenation and ventilation.

85. On arrival at the destination hospital, pretransport ventilator settings and appropriate alarm limits are set on the ventilator _____ (as soon as possible, after the patient has been stabilized from the transport).

86. During transport of mechanically ventilated patients, _____ is the only alternative in the event of ventilator failure.

87. When an aircraft is not pressurized, the patient's oxygenation status should be monitored with a _____ (pulse oximeter, capnography). Any arterial oxygen desaturation due to the high-altitude condition may be corrected by increasing the _____ (F_IO_2, frequency, tidal volume).

88. Steel oxygen cylinders should not be used where magnetic resonance imaging (MRI) is being done. Instead, aluminum oxygen cylinders are safe near the MRI source. _____ (TRUE/FALSE)

89. Most ventilators that are common in the ICU may be used safely near the MRI source. _____ (TRUE/FALSE)

CHAPTER 15

Critical Care Issues in Mechanical Ventilation

ACUTE LUNG INJURY AND ACUTE RESPIRATORY DISTRESS SYNDROME

1. Lung injuries occur during mechanical ventilation because the lungs in some critically ill patients are _____ (homogenous, nonhomogenous) in structure and they have _____ (similar, different) compliance and opening pressure requirements.

2. Repeated opening and closing of the alveoli during mechanical ventilation _____ (increases, decreases) the shearing force to the lungs.

3. When nonhomogenous lungs are ventilated by positive pressure, the _____ (compliant, noncompliant) units are opened and closed intermittently, while the _____ compliant, noncompliant) units suffer from overdistension.

4. The mortality rates of patients with ARDS are consistently between 40% and 50%. _____ (TRUE/FALSE)

5. Acute lung injury (ALI) and acute respiratory distress syndrome (ARDS) share all of the following clinical features *except*:

   A. $PaO_2/F_IO_2 \leq 300$ mm Hg regardless of PEEP level.

   B. acute onset.

   C. bilateral infiltrate.

   D. PCWP ≤ 18 mm Hg and without signs of left atrial hypertension.

6. The oxygenation threshold for _____ (ARDS, ALI) is $PaO_2/F_IO_2 \leq 300$ mm Hg.

7. The oxygenation threshold for _____ (ARDS, ALI) is $PaO_2/F_IO_2 \leq 200$ mm Hg.

8. If the bilateral infiltrates are due to _____ (ARDS, left-heart dysfunction or failure), the PCWP would be ≥ 18 mm Hg.

9. ALI, ARDS, and acute alveolar hypoventilation _____ (can, cannot) cause a significant decrease in PaO_2 *and* PaO_2/F_IO_2.

10. _____ (Direct, Indirect) injury to the lungs can lead to pathological abnormality in the intra-alveolar space and alveolar filling by edema, fibrin, collagen, neutrophilic aggregates, or blood.

11. Pneumonia, inhalation of toxins, and pulmonary contusion are some conditions associated with _____ (direct, indirect) lung injury.

12. _____ (Direct, Indirect) injury to the lungs primarily leads to microvascular congestion and interstitial edema, with relative sparing of the intra-alveolar spaces.

13. Sepsis, acute pancreatitis, and transfusion of blood products are some conditions related to _____ (direct, indirect) lung injury.

14. The current management strategy for ALI and ARDS is supportive care for _____ (infection control, nutritional supplement, oxygenation and ventilation).

15. Tachypnea, tachycardia, and mild hypoxemia are the _____ (early, late) clinical signs of ARDS.

16. An increasing $PaCO_2$ and development of severe respiratory acidosis usually _____ (precede, follow) a period of severe hypoxemia (i.e., low PaO_2/F_IO_2 ratio).

17. V/Q mismatch and intrapulmonary shunting are the leading causes of _____ (hypercapnia, hypoxemia) in patients with ARDS.

18. During the exudative phase of ALI and ARDS, chest radiographs typically reveal _____ (ipsilateral [on the same side], bilateral) infiltrates and alveolar opacities.

19. The radiographic signs of pulmonary edema caused by ARDS and congestive heart failure are _____ (similar, different).

20. Cardiomegaly, pleural effusions, and vascular redistribution are some signs of _____ (cardiogenic, noncardiogenic) pulmonary edema. The PCWP measurements should be _____ (normal, elevated) when pulmonary edema is caused by left-heart failure.

21. To protect the lungs from excessive airway pressures, the following traditional thresholds may be used as a guide: peak inspiratory pressures _____ (< 50 cm H_2O, < 70 cm H_2O), plateau pressures _____ (< 35 cm H_2O, < 50 cm H_2O), mean airway pressures _____ (< 30 cm H_2O, < 40 cm H_2O) and PEEP _____ (< 10 cm H_2O, < 5 cm H_2O).

22. In 2000, the ARDSNet recommended that the plateau pressure be kept _____ (< 20 cm H_2O, < 30 cm H_2O).

23. _____ (High, Low) airway pressure and _____ (high, low) tidal volume increase the risk for ARDS in patients receiving mechanical ventilation.

24. The airway pressure can be reduced by using a _____ (higher, lower) tidal volume during volume-controlled ventilation.

25. For patients with COPD, the peak inspiratory flow should be _____ (increased, decreased) to allow a longer expiratory time for adequate exhalation.

26. Complications of using _____ (high, low) tidal volume for mechanical ventilation include acute hypercapnia and respiratory acidosis, increased work of breathing, dyspnea, and atelectasis.

27. Permissive hypercapnia uses low _____ (peak inspiratory pressure, tidal volume) during volume-controlled ventilation and allows the _____ (PaO_2, $PaCO_2$) to rise above 50 mm Hg.

28. The tidal volume used in permissive hypercapnia is in the range of _____ (2 to 4 mL/kg, 4 to 7 mL/kg, 7 to 10 mL/kg).

29. To implement permissive hypercapnia, the _____ (peak inspiratory pressure, tidal volume) is titrated until the PIP is near the _____ (positive end-expiratory pressure, plateau pressure) measured before the low tidal volume procedure. Using the _____ (positive end-expiratory pressure, plateau pressure) as the target PIP avoids alveolar overdistention.

30. Permissive hypercapnia leads to an elevated $PaCO_2$, _____ (alkalosis, acidosis), and adverse effects on the CNS, intracranial pressure, or cardiovascular system.

31. The acidosis resulting from permissive hypercapnia may be returned to normal either by renal compensation over time or by neutralizing the acid with:

    A. carbonic acid.

    B. bicarbonate.

    C. tromethamine.

    D. B and C only.

32. _____ (Bicarbonate, Tromethamine) is preferred because it compensates for metabolic acidosis by directly decreasing the hydrogen ion concentration and indirectly _____ (increasing, decreasing) the carbon dioxide level.

33. For patients with ARDS, the lung units with low compliance require _____ (high, low) opening and sustaining pressures. These airway pressures can overstretch and injure the compliant normal lung units.

34. The detrimental effects of PEEP include all of the following *except*:

    A. decrease in peak inspiratory pressure.

    B. increase in pleural pressure and pulmonary vascular resistance.

    C. decrease in left-ventricular compliance.

    D. decrease in venous return, cardiac output, and systemic oxygen delivery.

35. In the management of patients with ARDS, the ARDSNet recommends _____ (pressure-controlled ventilation, volume-controlled ventilation) with a(n) _____ (A/C, SIMV) mode.

36. The ARDSNet also recommends keeping the P_{PLAT} _____ (<30 cm H_2O, <50 cm H_2O) with low tidal volume setting and using a combination of F_IO_2 and PEEP to keep O_2 saturation _____ (>88%, >92%, >95%).

37. Using the ARDSNet recommendation, for an F_IO_2 of 60% the initial accompanying PEEP should be _____ (8, 10, 12) cm H_2O.

38. A decremental recruitment maneuver is done to determine the _____ (peak pressure setting, mean airway pressure, optimal PEEP).

39. Different methods for the titration of optimal PEEP use the same criteria to determine the titration endpoints. _____ (TRUE/FALSE)

40. During the *initial* recruitment maneuver (Step 3 in Table 15-4 of textbook), the patient _____ (is, is not) sedated and _____ (does, does not) breathe spontaneously.

41. Immediately after the initial recruitment maneuver, the patient is placed on _____ (volume-controlled ventilation, pressure-controlled ventilation) at a PEEP of _____ (10, 15, 20) cm H_2O for a total pressure of _____ (15, 25, 35, 45) cm H_2O.

42. Following the initial recruitment maneuver, the F_IO_2 is decreased gradually by 5% to 20% until SpO_2 stabilizes between _____ (88% and 90%, 90% and 94%, 92% and 96%), and the PEEP is decreased gradually by _____ (2, 4, 6) cm H_2O increments every 15 to 20 minutes until the SpO_2 drops below 90%.

43. The optimal PEEP is the PEEP level _____ (precisely when the SpO_2 reaches 90%, immediately before the SpO_2 drops below 90%).

44. The final recruitment maneuver is done by using an F_IO_2 of _____ (40%, 100%) and _____ (PEEP, CPAP) of 40 cm H_2O for _____ (20, 30, 40) seconds.

45. A recruitment maneuver should be used on selected patients with severe _____ (pulmonary edema, heart failure) and who are most at risk of dying from refractory hypoxemia due to ALI or ARDS.

46. A recruitment maneuver can be done safely to patients with existing barotraumas, unstable hemodynamic status, presence of blebs or bullae on chest radiograph, and increased intracranial pressure. _____ (TRUE/FALSE)

47. Prone positioning is done by placing the patient in a _____ (face-up; face-down) position and the bed in a _____ (Trendelenberg, reverse Trendelenberg) position at 15 to 30 degrees. Since the patient is in a prone position, the majority of the _____ (upper, middle, lower) lobes are in an uppermost position.

48. Prone positioning reduces the opening pressure of the _____ (upper, middle, lower) lobes for better distribution of ventilation and a reduced transpulmonary pressure gradient.

49. The indication for prone positioning is patients who require a PEEP _____ (>5 cm H_2O, > 10 cm H_2O) and F_IO_2 _____ (≥40% ≥60%) to maintain supine oxygen saturation of ≥90%.

VENTILATOR-ASSOCIATED PNEUMONIA

50. By definition, ventilator-associated pneumonia (VAP) is a(n) _____ (existing, newly acquired) infection of the lung parenchyma that develops within _____ (24, 48) hours after intubation and initiation of mechanical ventilation.

51. Risk factors for VAP include long duration of mechanical ventilation and all of the following conditions *except*:

    A. advanced age.

    B. obesity.

    C. depressed level of consciousness.

    D. preexisting lung disease.

52. VAP is associated with fever, leukocytosis or leukopenia, and hemoptysis. _____ (TRUE/FALSE)

53. The radiographic signs of VAP include new or progressive infiltrates on chest radiography. _____ (TRUE/FALSE)

54. Methicillin-resistant *Staphylococcus aureus* (MRSA) is the predominant pathogen in VAP _____ (during the first 48 hours, from 3 to 7 days, for more than 7 days) following intubation and initiation of mechanical ventilation.

55. Which of the following is *not* a parameter in the modified clinical pulmonary infection score (CPIS)?

    A. Electrolytes

    B. Chest X-ray infiltrates

    C. PaO_2/F_IO_2

    D. Body temperature

56. To minimize the development of VAP, the head of bed should be elevated at an angle of _____ (10 to 20 degrees; 30 to 45 degrees) _____ (for 30 minutes every 4 hours, at all times), and the ventilator circuit should be changed _____ (every 3 days, when visibly soiled).

57. Sedation should be discontinued to allow weaning assessment and early extubation. _____ (TRUE/FALSE)

58. An endotracheal tube with a separate dorsal lumen above the cuff is designed for the primary purpose of _____ (lowering the cuff pressure, removing subglottic secretions).

59. Empiric _____ (antibacterial, antiviral, broad-spectrum) antibiotics are recommended for the treatment of VAP. These drugs are administered _____ (before, after) the pathogens are identified.

HYPOXIC-ISCHEMIC ENCEPHALOPATHY

60. Hypoxic-ischemic encephalopathy (HIE) is a condition caused by a severe lack of oxygen supply to the _____ (heart, brain, kidneys), leading to damage to the cells and neurons of the brain and spinal cord.

61. Which of the following is *not* a condition leading to HIE?

    A. Inadequate ventilation or oxygenation

    B. Inadequate perfusion

    C. Increase in cerebral perfusion pressure

    D. Decrease in cerebral perfusion pressure

62. Outline the mechanism of cerebral cellular injury starting from "energy failure" due to depletion of glucose and ATP stores.

    _____

    _____

    _____

63. Given: CPP = MAP – ICP. Cerebral perfusion pressure (CPP), Mean arterial pressure (MAP), Intracranial pressure (ICP).

    Perfusion-related conditions (e.g., cardiac arrest, severe hypotension) are conditions that cause a(n) _____ (direct, indirect) reduction in cerebral perfusion. Non-perfusion-related conditions (e.g., increase in intracranial pressure) cause a(n) _____ (direct, indirect) reduction in cerebral perfusion.

64. Diminished concentration, poor judgment or coordination, euphoria, and extreme lethargy are some signs of _____ (mild, severe) cerebral oxygen deprivation.

65. The critical threshold for CPP is from _____ (70 to 80 mm Hg, 90 to 110 mm Hg), and the mortality rate increases about 20% for each 10 mm Hg _____ (increase, decrease) in CPP from the threshold.

66. Following successful resuscitation, the long-term prognosis for patients who initially survive a cardiac arrest is excellent. _____ (TRUE/FALSE)

67. To manage severe hypotension due to cardiac arrest, all of the following should be done with the *exception* of:

    A. fluid.

    B. oxygen.

    C. beta agonists.

    D. vasodilators.

68. Blood loss is an example of _____ (absolute, relative) hypovolemia and the primary treatment is _____ (blood replacement, vasopressor drugs, antibiotics).

69. Septic shock is an example of _____ (absolute, relative) hypovolemia and the primary treatment is _____ (treatment of septicemia, blood replacement, vasopressor drugs).

70. Given: CPP = MAP – ICP. The CPP may become inadequate when the MAP is too _____ (high, low) or when the ICP is too _____ (high, low).

71. In clinical practice, ICP control is _____ (necessary, not necessary) because ICP tends to _____ (go over, stay below) its clinical threshold of 20 mm Hg under normal conditions.

72. The CPP can be maintained above the critical threshold of 20 mm Hg by raising the MAP with fluid support and _____ (vasodilators, vasopressors).

73. The systolic blood pressure should be kept above _____ (70 mm Hg, 90 mm Hg, 110 mm Hg) as soon as it is feasible, since early hypotension is associated with increased morbidity and mortality following severe brain injury.

74. An increase in ICP can _____ (increase, decrease) the CPP and blood supply to the brain.

75. A CT or MRI scan, EEG, ultrasound, and an evoked potential test may be used to evaluate the severity of anatomic and physiologic changes in the brain and spinal cord. _____ (TRUE/FALSE)

76. Sustained hypothermia is a treatment option for HIE because this procedure _____ (provides a higher oxygen saturation at any F_1O_2, reduces oxygen consumption and effects of cerebral hypoxia).

TRAUMATIC BRAIN INJURY

77. Traumatic brain injury (TBI) may be caused by all of the following conditions *except*:

   A. severe hypoxia.

   B. motor vehicle crashes.

   C. sports-related injuries.

   D. explosive blasts and combat injuries.

78. Almost 100% of patients with a severe head injury become permanently disabled in performing some daily functions. _____ (TRUE/FALSE)

79. Under normal condition, the brain occupies _____ (75 to 80%, 85 to 90%) of the intracranial compartment. In addition, the brain has a very _____ (high, low) compliance and _____ (can, cannot) tolerate significant rapid volume expansion.

80. Significant volume expansion within a rigid skull will cause the intracranial pressure (ICP) to _____ (increase, decrease). This condition results in a(n) _____ (increased, decreased) cerebral perfusion pressure and cerebral perfusion.

81. The normal ICP is 8 to 12 mm Hg and its clinical normal is up to _____ (16 mm Hg, 20 mm Hg, 24 mm Hg).

82. A suboptimal CPP is defined as a measurement of less than _____ (70 mm Hg, 90 mm Hg), and this condition can cause cerebral hypoxia or ischemia and death.

83. Brain injury acquired at the moment of impact is called _____ (primary, secondary) injury.

84. _____ (Primary, Secondary) injury to the brain may be due to an increase in intracranial pressure (ICP) and decrease in CPP and cerebral blood flow.

85. Brain injury can occur when the brain makes contact with the inside of the skull _____ (quickly, slowly).

86. A severe blow to the skull is an example of _____ (acceleration, deceleration) brain injury.

87. The skull falling on concrete is an example of _____ (acceleration, deceleration) brain injury.

88. In explosive blasts, brain injury occurs when the _____ (sound wave, pressure wave) passes through the brain, directly causing disruption to the brain function.

89. Brain herniation occurs as a result of increased _____ (CPP, ICP).

90. Brain injury can occur when the brain _____ (passes through the dural openings, makes contact with the prominent edges of the dural openings).

91. Transtentorial herniation is a type of brain injury that causes the _____ (upward, downward) displacement of the medial aspect of the temporal lobe (uncus) through the tentorial notch by a mass above.

92. _____ (Unilateral, Bilateral) dilated pupil is a classic sign of transtentorial herniation of the brain.

93. Mild TBI has a Glasgow coma scale (GCS) score of _____ (6 to 8, 10 to 12, 13 to 14).

94. A GCS score of 3 to 8 indicates _____ (mild, moderate, severe) brain injury.

95. The three parameters of the Glasgow coma scale are:

    A. eye opening, motor response, verbal response.

    B. hand grip, head lift, eye opening.

    C. head lift, verbal response, vital signs.

    D. motor response, head lift, vital signs.

96. In the management of severe TBI, all of the following procedures should be done *except*:

    A. protect airway.

    B. provide eucapnic ventilation and adequate oxygenation.

    C. correct hypovolemia and hypotension.

    D. perform and evaluate chest radiography.

97. To prevent hypotension, the _____ (diastolic, systolic) blood pressure should be kept above 90 mm Hg.

98. To reduce cerebral blood flow and intracranial pressure, the $PaCO_2$ may be titrated to a level as low as _____ (20 torr, 26 torr, 33 torr) during the first _____ (8, 12, 24) hours of mechanical ventilation.

CHAPTER 16

Weaning from Mechanical Ventilation

DEFINITION OF WEANING SUCCESS AND FAILURE

1. Weaning success is defined as absence of ventilatory support _____ (12, 24, 48) hours following extubation.

2. The time needed to wean patients with medical conditions is generally _____ (longer, shorter) because they have _____ (more, fewer) coexisting medical problems.

3. Weaning in progress describes the patients who _____ (are, are not) extubated and receive ventilatory support by noninvasive ventilation (NIV).

4. Weaning failure is defined as failure of the spontaneous breathing trial (SBT) or the need for reintubation within _____ (12, 24, 48) following extubation.

PATIENT CONDITION PRIOR TO WEANING

5. Before a weaning trial is begun, the patient should be fully recovered from the condition resulting in ventilatory support and be able to assume _____ (oxygenation, spontaneous breathing).

6 to 8. Match the conditions that may hinder weaning success with the respective examples. Use each answer only *once*.

CONDITION	EXAMPLE
6. _____ Patient/pathophysiologic	A. Nutritional deficit, pH imbalance
7. _____ Cardiac/circulatory	B. Fever, infection, sleep deprivation
8. _____ Dietary/acid-base/ electrolytes	C. Arrhythmias, abnormal blood pressures, hypotension

WEANING CRITERIA

9. Weaning criteria are used to evaluate the:

    A. readiness of a patient to begin the weaning trial.

    B. likelihood of weaning success.

    C. readiness for extubation.

    D. A and B only.

10. Weaning is more likely to succeed if a patient meets _____ (one or two, most) of the weaning criteria.

11 to 16. Write in the normal value or normal range for each of the following *ventilatory* weaning criteria.

VENTILATORY WEANING CRITERIA	NORMAL VALUE/RANGE
11. Spontaneous breathing trial	Tolerates _____ to _____ min
12. $PaCO_2$	<_____ mm Hg with normal pH
13. Vital capacity (VC)	>_____ mL/kg
14. Spontaneous V_T	>_____ mL/kg
15. Spontaneous f	<_____ /min
16. f/V_T	<_____ breaths/min/L

17 to 22. Write in the normal value for each of the following *oxygenation* weaning criteria.

OXYGENATION WEANING CRITERIA	NORMAL VALUE
17. PaO_2 (without PEEP)	_____ mm Hg at F_IO_2 up to 0.4
18. PaO_2 (with PEEP <8 cm H_2O)	_____ mm Hg at F_IO_2 up to 0.4
19. SaO_2	_____ at F_IO_2 up to 0.4
20. PaO_2/F_IO_2 (P/F)	_____ mm Hg
21. Q_S/Q_T	_____ %
22. $P(A-a)O_2$	_____ mm Hg at F_IO_2 of 1.0

23 to 24. Write in the normal value or normal range for each of the following *pulmonary reserve* weaning criteria.

PULMONARY RESERVE WEANING CRITERIA	NORMAL VALUE/RANGE
23. Vital capacity	_____ mL/kg
24. Maximum inspiratory pressure	_____ to _____ cm H_2O in 20 sec

25 to 26. Write in the normal value for each of the following *pulmonary measurement* weaning criteria.

PULMONARY MEASUREMENT WEANING CRITERIA	NORMAL VALUE
25. Static compliance	_____ mL/cm H_2O
26. V_D/V_T	_____ %

27. The partial pressure of carbon dioxide in the arterial blood ($PaCO_2$) is the most reliable indicator of a patient's _____ (oxygenation, acid-base, ventilatory) status.

28. Weaning from mechanical ventilation should be attempted only when the $PaCO_2$ is between _____ and _____ mm Hg with a(n) _____ (acidotic, compensated, alkalotic) pH. The $PaCO_2$ may be _____ (higher, lower) for chronic obstructive pulmonary disease (COPD) patients.

29. Explain why it is desirable to allow the patient to breathe spontaneously for 3 minutes prior to measuring the VC and spontaneous tidal volume.

_____

_____

30. The _____ (tidal volume, vital capacity) measurement is effort-dependent. Valid measurements of this weaning parameter _____ (require, do not require) proper explanation and coaching.

31. For a successful weaning outcome, the spontaneous respiratory frequency should be _____ (more than, less than) 35 breaths/min while the corresponding $PaCO_2$ should be _____ (more than, less than) 50 mm Hg.

32. A _____ (fast, slow) breathing pattern is a sign of respiratory distress and it reflects _____ (good, poor) readiness for the weaning trial.

33. The patient's spontaneous resting minute volume should be _____ (more, less) than 10 L/min for a successful weaning outcome, because a _____ (high, low) minute ventilation requirement implies that the work of breathing is excessive.

34. An excessive minute volume requirement may be caused by a(n) _____ (increased, decreased) carbon dioxide production secondary to metabolic _____ (acidosis, alkalosis), or a(n) _____ (increased, decreased) metabolic rate or deadspace-to-tidal-volume ratio.

35. Causes of a(n) _____ (increased, decreased) carbon dioxide production include extensive burn injuries, an elevated body temperature, and sometimes overfeeding, especially with _____ (fat, carbohydrate) dietary supplements.

36. PaO_2 and SpO_2 measurements _____ (do, do not) reflect the true oxygenation status of patients with anemia or increased levels of dysfunctional hemoglobins. Under these conditions, _____ (arterial $PaCO_2$, arterial oxygen content, arterial pH) should be used to evaluate a patient's oxygenation status.

37. The physiologic shunt (Q_S/Q_T) is used to estimate how much _____ (ventilation, pulmonary perfusion) is wasted. An increased Q_S/Q_T usually leads to _____ (hypercapnia, hypoxemia, acidosis).

38. A patient has the following oxygen content measurements: CcO_2 = 20 vol%, CaO_2 = 18 vol%, CvO_2 = 13 vol%. The calculated Q_S/Q_T is about _____ and it reflects _____ shunting.

    A. 10%, mild

    B. 29%, significant

    C. 35%, severe

    D. 65%, severe

39. A patient is being assessed for a weaning trial and the blood gas parameters are as follows: F_IO_2 = 100%, P_AO_2 = 650 mm Hg, PaO_2 = 200 mm Hg. The calculated $P(A-a)O_2$ is _____ and the estimated physiologic shunt is _____.

    A. 450 mm Hg, 10%

    B. 450 mm Hg, 18%

    C. 850 mm Hg, 10%

    D. 85 mm Hg, 18%

40. On 100% F_IO_2, every 50 mm Hg difference in $P(A-a)O_2$ approximates _____ (1, 2, 5) % physiologic shunt.

41. The arterial oxygen tension to inspired oxygen concentration (PaO_2/F_IO_2) index is a simplified method for estimating the degree of _____ (deadspace ventilation, ventilation/perfusion mismatch, intrapulmonary shunt).

42. A PaO_2/F_IO_2 index of 150 mm Hg or _____ (higher, lower) is indicative of normal physiologic shunt and compatible to a successful weaning trial.

43. Vital capacity (VC) and maximum inspiratory pressure (MIP) are two weaning criteria that are used to reflect a patient's _____ ($PaCO_2$, PaO_2, pulmonary reserve).

44. Explain why proper explanation and coaching is important before obtaining the VC and MIP measurements.

    _____

    _____

45. VC measures the maximum amount of lung volume that the patient can exhale following _____ (tidal inspiration, maximal inspiration).

46. For a more successful weaning outcome, the patient should have a VC of greater than _____ mL/kg.

47. MIP is the amount of _____ (positive, negative) pressure that a patient can generate in 20 sec when inspiring against an _____ (opened, occluded) pressure manometer.

48. For a more successful weaning outcome, the patient should be able to generate an MIP of greater than _____ cm H_2O.

49. A patient's work of breathing is increased in conditions of _____ (high, low) compliance, _____ (high, low) airway resistance, and _____ (high, low) V_D/V_T ratio.

50. The static lung compliance is calculated by dividing the patient's tidal volume by the difference in the _____ (peak airway, plateau) pressure and the PEEP.

51. A static compliance (C_{ST}) value of 30 mL/cm H_2O or _____ (greater, less) is consistent with a readiness to begin the weaning process.

52. The airway resistance is calculated by dividing the difference in the _____ (peak airway, plateau) pressure and the _____ (plateau pressure, PEEP) by the constant inspiratory flow.

53. _____ (PEEP, Pressure-controlled ventilation, Pressure support ventilation) is effective in reducing the circuit and airflow resistance during spontaneous breathing.

54. The V_D/V_T ratio estimates the volume of each breath that is being perfused by pulmonary circulation. _____ (TRUE/FALSE)

55. The blood gases and related parameters of a patient are as follows: pH = 7.43, $PaCO_2$ = 40 mm Hg, PaO_2 = 80 mm Hg, P_ECO_2 = 30 mm Hg. What portion of the tidal volume is considered wasted (deadspace) ventilation?

    A. 25%

    B. 50%

    C. 75%

    D. Insufficient data to calculate answer

RAPID SHALLOW BREATHING INDEX (RSBI)

56. For a successful weaning outcome, the respiratory frequency to tidal volume (f/V_T) ratio (rapid shallow breathing index or RSBI) should be _____ (100, 120, 150, 200) breaths/min/L or lower.

57. Shallow breathing leads to _____ (efficient, inefficient) ventilation because the anatomic deadspace volume contributes to a _____ (larger, lower) V_D/V_T ratio when the tidal volume is reduced.

58. A high f/V_T ratio indicates _____ (efficient, inefficient) ventilation. Therefore, a successful weaning outcome should have an f/V_T ratio of _____ (more than, less than) 100 breaths/min/L.

59. Describe the procedure to measure the f/V_T ratio.

    _____

    _____

    _____

    _____

60. A patient who is being considered for weaning has these measurements obtained during spontaneous breathing: V_E = 4.2 L/min, f = 16/min. What is the patient's f/V_T ratio? Does the ratio predict a successful weaning outcome?

   A. 38; successful weaning outcome

   B. 61; successful weaning outcome

   C. 38; unsuccessful weaning outcome

   D. 61; unsuccessful weaning outcome

WEANING PROCEDURE

61. A spontaneous breathing trial (SBT) is done by using a spontaneous breathing mode via the ventilator or T-tube (Brigg's adaptor) for up to _____ (10, 30, 60) minutes.

62. During SBT, oxygen and low-level pressure support may be used to supplement oxygenation and augment spontaneous breathing. _____ (TRUE/FALSE)

63. For a successful SBT, the patient _____ (should, should not) have a rapid shallow breathing pattern.

64. Patients who fail the SBT usually do so within the first _____ (5 to 10, 10 to 20, 20 to 30) minutes of SBT.

65. T-tube, CPAP, or automatic tube compensation may be used during the SBT. _____ (TRUE/FALSE)

66. The SBT may last for up to _____ minutes.

67. The SBT may be supplemented with pressure support for up to _____ cm H_2O for adults and _____ cm H_2O for pediatrics.

68. SIMV _____ (is, is not) recommended as a stand-alone mode for weaning.

69. The SIMV frequency is _____ (increased, decreased) by _____ (1 to 3, 3 to 5) breaths-per-minute increments as the patient's spontaneous breathing effort improves.

70. Pressure support ventilation should be set *initially* between _____ (5 to 15, 10 to 20) cm H_2O until the tidal volume is _____ (10 to 15, 10 to 20) mL/kg or the spontaneous frequency is _____ (15, 25, 35) per minute or less.

71. As the patient's spontaneous breathing efforts improve, the pressure support level is withdrawn by _____ (1 to 3, 3 to 6, 6 to 9) cm H_2O increments until a level of close to _____ (1, 5, 10) cm H_2O is reached.

72. Once the PSV reaches _____ (1, 5, 10) cm H_2O, the patient may be extubated when the blood gases and vital signs are satisfactory.

73. When the patient fails the SBT, it usually occurs within _____ (30, 60, 120) minutes.

74 to 82. Complete the thresholds for the 9 criteria that are related to SBT *failure*.

74. PaO_2 ≤_____ mm Hg on F_IO_2 ≥50%

75. SaO_2 <_____ on F_IO_2 ≥50%

76. $PaCO_2$ >_____ mm Hg or an increase in $PaCO_2$ >8 mm Hg from baseline

77. pH   <_____ or a decrease in pH ≥0.07 from baseline

78. f/V_T >_____ breaths/min/L

79. spontaneous f   >_____ /min or increase by ≥50% from baseline

80. heart rate   >_____ beats/min or increase by ≥20% from baseline

81. Systolic BP (high)   >_____ mm Hg or increase by ≥20% from baseline

82. Systolic BP (low)   <_____ mm Hg

83. Weaning with PSV is done by starting the pressure support level at 5 to 15 cm H_2O and adjusting it gradually (up to _____ (20, 30, 40) cm H_2O) until a desired spontaneous V_T (10 to 15 mL/kg) or spontaneous frequency is reached, typically 25/min or less.

84. Automatic tube compensation (ATC) is used to reduce the airflow resistance imposed by the _____ (lungs, large airways, artificial airway).

85. Volume support (VS) and volume-assured pressure support (VAPS) are a form of _____ (noninvasive ventilation, pressure support ventilation) that "guarantees" a preset tidal volume.

86. In VS, the pressure support level is _____ (based on the patient's effort, adjusted automatically by the ventilator) to achieve the target tidal volume.

87. In VAPS, it guarantees a preset tidal volume by incorporating _____ (inspiratory, expiratory) pressure support ventilation with conventional volume-assisted ventilation.

88. In mandatory minute ventilation (MMV), the ventilator adjusts the _____ (SIMV frequency, SIMV volume) automatically to achieve the target minute ventilation.

89. In airway pressure-release ventilation (APRV), the _____ (peak pressure, plateau, tidal volume) is determined by the pressure gradient between the airway pressure and the release pressure.

90. In APRV, _____ (inhalation, exhalation) occurs during pressure release and _____ (inhalation, exhalation) occurs when the pressure returns to the airway pressure.

WEANING PROTOCOL

91. A weaning protocol should be used as prescribed regardless of the patient's disease process or condition. _____ (TRUE/FALSE)

92. Weaning protocols are _____ (suggested, mandated) guidelines for practitioners to carry out the weaning process.

93. Based on the weaning protocol described in the textbook, all of the following conditions must be met for consideration of a weaning attempt *except*:

    A. presence of inspiratory effort.

    B. hemodynamic stability.

    C. PaO_2 / F_IO_2 <150 mm Hg.

    D. little or no sedation required.

94. Prior to measuring the data for RSBI, the patient should be breathing spontaneously for at least _____ (1, 3, 5, 10) minutes or until a stable breathing pattern is reached.

95. For a successful and sustainable weaning outcome, the patient must be able to tolerate the SBT for _____ (10, 20, 30) minutes without vital sign or hemodynamic instability.

SIGNS OF WEANING FAILURE

96. The weaning process should be _____ (continued, stopped) if the patient shows signs of muscle fatigue, hemodynamic instability, or ventilatory failure.

97. A patient may _____ (hyperventilate, hypoventilate) as a result of hypoxia, pain, anxiety, or inappropriate ventilator settings. When this condition occurs, the $PaCO_2$ would _____ (increase, decrease) and the therapist should _____ (decrease the level of ventilatory support immediately, assess the patient and find the cause for hyperventilation).

98. All of the following are early signs of weaning failure *except*:

    A. eucapnic ventilation.

    B. use of accessory muscles.

    C. paradoxical abdominal movements.

    D. diaphoresis.

99 to 101. Complete the following indicators of weaning failure.

INDICATOR	EXAMPLE
99. Blood gases	Increasing $PaCO_2$ to _____ mm Hg
	Decreasing pH to _____
	Decreasing PaO_2 to _____ mm Hg
	Decreasing SaO_2 or SpO_2 to _____%
	Decreasing PaO_2 / F_IO_2 to _____ mm Hg
100. Vital signs	Changing blood pressures by _____ mm Hg systolic or _____ mm Hg diastolic
	Increasing heart rate by _____/min, or _____/min

101. Respiratory parameters

Decreasing V_T to _____ mL

Increasing f to _____/min

Increasing (f/V_T) ratio to _____ breaths/min/L

Decreasing MIP to _____ cm H_2O

Decreasing C_{ST} to _____ cm H_2O/L

Increasing V_D/V_T to _____%

CAUSES OF WEANING FAILURE

102. List the three major causes of weaning failure.

_____

_____

_____

103. To minimize the effect on airflow resistance, a size _____ (6, 8) or larger ET tube should be used for adults because its cross-sectional area is similar to that of an adult _____ (trachea, bronchus, glottis).

104. Another strategy to reduce the airflow resistance during mechanical ventilation is to cut the ET tube to about _____ (1 cm, 1 in., 2 in.) from the patient's lips or nares.

105. The section of ET tube that is cut should be _____ (discarded, displayed prominently). Explain.

_____

_____

106. Other causes of increased airway resistance during mechanical ventilation include all of the following conditions *except*:

   A. kinking of ET tube.

   B. secretions in ET tube.

   C. use of pulse oximeter.

   D. use of heat-and-moisture exchanger.

107. _____ (High, Low) lung or thoracic compliance makes lung expansion difficult, and it is a major contributing factor to respiratory muscle fatigue and weaning failure.

108. List at least three clinical conditions that may lead to a decreased C_{ST}.

_____

_____

_____

109. List at least three clinical conditions that may lead to a decreased *dynamic* compliance.

_____

_____

_____

110. Given: work of breathing = P_{TP} (transpulmonary pressure) x V_T (tidal volume). Based on this equation, the work of breathing is increased when the transpulmonary pressure is _____ (increased, decreased).

111. The transpulmonary pressure is increased in conditions of _____ (high, low) compliance or _____ (high, low) airway resistance.

112. Persistent increase of the transpulmonary pressure may lead to respiratory muscle fatigue and eventual ventilatory failure. _____ (TRUE/FALSE)

113. Respiratory muscle dysfunction may be due to all of the following conditions *except*:

    A. respiratory muscular atrophy due to muscle disuse.

    B. excessive nutritional intake.

    C. low oxygen delivery.

    D. electrolyte imbalance.

114. Describe two methods that may improve the functions of the respiratory muscles and diaphragms after prolonged mechanical ventilation and muscle disuse.

_____

_____

TERMINAL WEANING

115. Terminal weaning is defined as the _____ (withholding, withdrawal) of mechanical ventilation, which results in the death of a patient.

116. A patient's informed consent means that the patient agrees to have the life-sustaining devices removed and he/she understands the potential consequences, including _____ (vegetative state, death).

117. Discussions on a patient's informed consent should be done _____ (during the physician rounds, over a period of time). Explain why.

_____

_____

118. Terminal weaning may be justified if medical intervention is futile or _____ (hopeful, hopeless).

119. During terminal weaning, adequate sedatives and analgesics should be provided to patient for control of anxiety and pain. _____ (TRUE/FALSE)

CHAPTER 17

Neonatal Mechanical Ventilation

INTUBATION

1. In addition to an Apgar score of 3 or less obtained immediately after delivery, intubation of a neonate should be considered in all of the following conditions *except*:

   A. ineffective bag/mask ventilation.

   B. presence of thick meconium on delivery.

   C. premature rupture of amniotic membrane.

   D. endotracheal (ET) administration of epinephrine or surfactant is indicated.

2. Intubation is also indicated in the presence of _____ (obstructive lesions, restrictive defects), such as Pierre-Robin syndrome, tracheomalacia, tracheal web, tracheal stenosis, laryngeal paralysis, and extrinsic masses.

3. Other indications of ET intubation may include all of the following *except*:

   A. removal of secretions.

   B. administration of oxygen.

   C. mechanical ventilation.

   D. collection of tracheal specimens.

4. The Apgar scores range from 0 to _____ and it is usually done _____ (1, 5, 1 and 5) min after birth.

5. Apgar scoring stops if the score is _____ (5, 7, 9) or higher in 5 min. If this minimum score is not obtained, scoring continues every 5 min up to _____ (10, 20, 30, 60) min.

6. Immediately after delivery, a neonate shows the following signs: heart rate of 110/min, irregular and shallow respiratory effort, well-flexed muscle tone, grimace on stimulation, and pink body but blue extremities. The total Apgar score for this assessment is _____ points. What are the individual scores for these five criteria?

_____

_____

_____

_____

_____

7. Use laryngoscope blade size _____ for most term newborns, size _____ for preemies, and size _____ for micropreemies.

8 to 10. Match the weights (gestational ages) with the appropriate ET tube sizes. Use only *three* answers.

WEIGHT (GESTATIONAL AGE)	TUBE SIZE (MM I.D.)
8. _____ Below 1000 g (less than 28 weeks)	A. 1.5
9. _____ 1000–2000 g (28–34 weeks)	B. 2.5
10. _____ 2000–3000 g (34–38 weeks)	C. 3.0
	D. 3.5
	E. 4.0

11. Each intubation attempt should be limited to less than _____ (10, 20, 30) sec to minimize hypoxia. It should be stopped sooner if the patient's condition dictates.

12. Describe the method to minimize hypoxia between prolonged intubation attempts.

_____

_____

_____

13. In addition to the vocal cord marking on the ET tube, a rule to estimate the depth of intubation in centimeters (cm) is to add _____ (3, 6, 9) to the infant's body weight in kilograms (kg).

SURFACTANT REPLACEMENT THERAPY

14. The primary cause of respiratory distress syndrome in the premature neonate is _____ .

15. Surfactant is a naturally occurring substance composed mainly of several _____ (sugars, carbohydrates, lipids, proteins).

16. About 90% of the surfactant is composed of _____, with phosphatidylcholine (PC) comprising 85% of the total amount.

17. About 60% of the PC is dipalmitoyl phosphatidylcholine (DPPC), a substance that allows surfactant to _____ (increase, lower) the surface tension.

18. Surfactant is most effective when given by _____ (aerosol administration, intravenous administration, direct instillation) into the _____ (systemic circulation, trachea).

19. _____ (Prophylactic, Therapeutic) administration of surfactant is indicated for those infants who are at a high risk of developing respiratory distress syndrome.

20. Based on the indications for prophylactic use of surfactant, the following condition must be met:

    A. birth weight less than 1250 g.

    B. gestational age at or less than 26 weeks.

    C. PaO_2/P_AO_2 less than 0.22.

    D. all of the above.

21. _____ (Prophylactic, Therapeutic) administration of surfactant is given when the neonate shows signs of respiratory distress syndrome.

22. Therapeutic or rescue administration of surfactant is indicated in infants with all of the following signs *except*:

    A. respiratory distress syndrome.

    B. progressive hypoxemia.

    C. ground glass appearance on chest radiograph.

    D. hyperventilation.

23. Respiratory distress syndrome is present when all of the following clinical signs are observed with the *exception* of:

    A. respiratory alkalosis.

    B. grunting.

    C. nasal flaring.

    D. chest retractions.

24. Surfaxin® is a _____ (natural, synthetic) surfactant. Survanta®, Infasurf®, and Alveofact® are naturally produced from _____ (sheep, pig, cow) lung tissue. Curosurf® is produced from _____ (sheep, pig, cow) lung tissue.

25. Surfactant replacement therapy has been used successfully to reduce the severity of _____ (respiratory distress syndrome, cystic fibrosis, meconium aspiration syndrome) and the incidence of some related cardiopulmonary complications.

26. Surfactant replacement therapy _____ (does, does not) work on all patients, and it has been implicated in the development of _____ (pulmonary hypertension, intraventricular hemorrhage, interstitial emphysema) in some neonates.

27. The dosage and frequency of administering Surfaxin®, Survanta®, Infasurf®, Alveofact®, and Curosurf® are the same. _____ (TRUE/FALSE)

NASAL CPAP

28. Nasal continuous positive airway pressure (N-CPAP) reduces V/Q mismatch by _____ (increasing, decreasing) the functional residual capacity and _____ (increasing, reducing) intrapulmonary shunting.

29. Along with surfactant administration, N-CPAP has been used successfully in many very-low-birth-weight infants and those with acute respiratory failure. _____ (TRUE/FALSE)

30. The initial N-CPAP settings for most infants range from _____ (1 to 4 cm H_2O, 4 to 7 cm H_2O, 7 to 10 cm H_2O) with flow rates from _____ (1 to 3 LPM, 3 to 5 LPM, 5 to 10 LPM).

BASIC PRINCIPLES OF NEONATAL VENTILATION

31. In pressure-controlled ventilation, a preset _____ (pressure, CPAP, PEEP) is used to deliver the tidal volume.

32. The tidal volumes delivered by pressure-controlled ventilation are dependent on the:

    A. patient's compliance.

    B. airflow resistance.

    C. pressure setting.

    D. all of the above.

33. In conditions of _____ (increasing, decreasing) compliance or _____ (increasing, decreasing) airway resistance, a higher peak inspiratory pressure is needed to maintain the same tidal volume.

34. When pressure-controlled ventilation is used, the delivered tidal volume _____ (increases, decreases) as the patient's respiratory condition improves. Explain why.

    _____

    _____

35. The peak inspiratory pressure setting during pressure-controlled ventilation should be reduced as the patient's compliance is _____ (increased, decreased) or the airway resistance is _____ (increased, decreased). Explain why.

    _____

    _____

36. In volume-controlled ventilation, the _____ (tidal volume, peak inspiratory pressure) is set by the therapist.

37. The tidal volumes delivered by volume-controlled ventilation are normally _____ (rather stable, highly irregular).

38. When volume-controlled ventilation is used, the peak inspiratory pressure _____ (increases, decreases) in conditions of decreasing compliance or increasing airflow resistance.

39. In volume-controlled ventilation, a(n) _____ (increasing, decreasing) peak inspiratory pressure may be a sign of increasing compliance or decreasing airflow resistance.

40. Inspiratory time (sec) multiplied by flow rate (mL/sec) approximates the _____ (pressure support level, vital capacity, tidal volume, peak inspiratory pressure).

41. Compressible volume is defined as the portion of ventilator volume that is _____ (added to, unaccounted for) and is within the ventilator circuit and humidifier during the inspiratory phase.

42. To minimize volume loss caused by expansion of the ventilator circuit, the circuit should have a _____ (high, low) compression factor.

43. Ideal ventilator circuits should have a _____ (high, low) compression factor so that the patient may receive the largest tidal volume possible from the ventilator.

44. To minimize volume loss within the humidifier, the humidifier used in a neonatal ventilator should also have a _____ (high, low) compressible volume.

45. Condensation or "rain-out" in the ventilator circuit occurs because the temperature _____ (increases, drops) as the gas moves from the humidifier through the patient circuit.

46. What are three potential problems when the water accumulates in the ventilator circuit?

    _____

    _____

    _____

47. A water trap placed inline on the _____ (inspiratory, expiratory) side of the ventilator circuit helps to prevent the problems caused by water accumulated in the circuit.

48. Heated wire may be placed inside the _____ (inspiratory, expiratory) tubing to reduce _____ (humidity deficit, condensation) in the ventilator circuit.

49. Premature shutdown (power off) of the heated wire may occur if the distal temperature probe is placed at the patient connection _____ (inside, outside) a heated incubator. Explain why.

    _____

    _____

50. To prevent premature shutdown (power off) of the heated wire, the temperature probe should be placed:

    A. outside the inlet to the incubator.

    B. inside the incubator.

    C. at the ET tube adaptor.

    D. inside the expiratory tubing.

INITIATION OF NEONATAL VENTILATORY SUPPORT

51. Indications for neonatal ventilatory support is based on the following general guidelines *except*:

    A. heart rate.

    B. apnea.

    C. hypercapnia.

    D. hypoxemia.

52. A physician wants to increase the tidal volume delivered to the neonate via pressure-controlled ventilation. This adjustment can be done by:

    A. increasing the pressure limit.

    B. increasing the tidal volume.

    C. decreasing the flow rate.

    D. decreasing the inspiratory time.

53. Which of the following is *not* a primary function of mechanical ventilation?

    A. Support of ventilatory failure

    B. Oxygenation

    C. Removal of carbon dioxide

    D. Correction of metabolic acidosis

54. The initial pressure setting on the ventilator should be slightly higher for neonates with _____ (high, low) compliance.

55. For infants with pulmonary air leak, the initial pressure setting on the ventilator should be slightly _____ (higher, lower) along with a _____ (higher, lower) frequency.

56 to 63. Complete the *initial* settings for neonatal ventilation based on normal or low compliance.

PARAMETER	NORMAL COMPLIANCE	LOW COMPLIANCE
56. PIP	_____ to _____ cm H_2O	_____ to _____ cm H_2O
57. PEEP	_____ to _____ cm H_2O	up to _____ cm H_2O
58. V_T	_____ to _____ mL/kg	_____ to _____ mL/kg
59. Frequency	_____ to _____ /min	Up to _____ /min (especially with air leak)
60. Flow rate	_____ to _____ L/min	_____ to _____ L/min
61. I time	_____ to _____ sec	Change according to frequency to maintain an I:E ratio of _____
62. I:E ratio	_____ to _____	At least _____
63. F_IO_2	_____	_____

64. During pressure-controlled ventilation, the inspiratory time and flow rate are set at 0.5 sec and 6 L/min, respectively. What is the estimated tidal volume?

    A. 12 mL

    B. 30 mL

    C. 50 mL

    D. Insufficient information to calculate answer

65. The initial F_IO_2 setting on a neonatal ventilator should be adjusted gradually to keep the patient pink while keeping the SpO2 from _____ (85 to 90%, 90 to 95%, 95 to 100%).

66. On those neonatal ventilators without a frequency control, the frequency is adjusted in this order:

    A. inspiratory time, expiratory time, flow.

    B. expiratory time, inspiratory time, flow.

    C. flow, inspiratory time, expiratory time.

    D. flow, expiratory time, inspiratory time.

67. A shorter inspiratory time may be necessary when the frequency setting on a neonatal ventilator is _____ (high, low) or in conditions of _____ (air trapping, air leak).

68. Using the neonate's body weight as a guide, _____ (3, 5, 8) mL/kg is the suggested tidal volume with a range of _____ (2 to 4, 3 to 7, 7 to 9) mL/kg.

69. The normal umbilical arterial blood gas values for neonates are: PO_2 _____ mm Hg, $PaCO_2$ _____ to _____ mm Hg, and pH _____ to _____.

70. For capillary samples, a _____ (higher, lower) PO_2 than arterial blood sample is expected and considered acceptable.

HIGH FREQUENCY VENTILATION (HFV)

71. High frequency ventilation (HFV) is a technique of ventilation that delivers _____ (large, normal, small) tidal volumes at very high frequencies.

72. How does HFV affect the peak inspiratory pressure and influence the incidence of barotrauma?

    _____

    _____

73. The use of HFV is often limited to those situations in which _____ (spontaneous ventilation, conventional mechanical ventilation, pressure support ventilation) has failed.

74. HFV appears to be most useful in treating _____ and pneumonia.

75. The frequencies generated by high frequency ventilators are measured in Hertz or cycles/min. One Hertz equals 1 cycle/sec or _____ cycles/min.

76. The major types of high frequency ventilators are categorized by the _____ of ventilation and the method with which the _____ is delivered.

77. High frequency positive pressure ventilation (HFPPV) delivers _____ (conventional, jet, pulsating) ventilatory breaths at frequencies between _____ and _____ breaths/min.

78. Describe the general indication of HFPPV.

_____

_____

79. In patients with severely noncompliant lungs, a high respiratory frequency may help to _____ (increase, decrease) the pressure requirement for the delivery of an adequate tidal volume.

80. Given: mPaw = [(f × I time / 60) × (PIP − PEEP)] + PEEP

   From the equation shown above, the mean airway pressure (mPaw) is _____ (directly, inversely) related to the respiratory frequency (f). Therefore, at high respiratory frequency settings, HFPPV tends to _____ (increase, decrease) the mPaw, risk of barotrauma, and cardiac compromise.

81. A high frequency jet ventilator (HFJV) delivers a high pressure _____ (tidal volume, pulse of gas) to the patient airway via a special adaptor attached to the ET tube.

82. HFJV operates at frequencies between _____ and _____/min or _____ and _____ Hz.

83. The indications for using HFJV include severe pulmonary disease that is complicated by all of the following *except*:

   A. pulmonary hypotension.

   B. air leaks.

   C. pulmonary hypoplasia.

   D. restrictive lung disease.

84. High frequency jet ventilation is used:

   A. after conventional ventilation has failed.

   B. to provide intrapulmonary percussion.

   C. in tandem with conventional mechanical ventilation.

   D. for premises with respiratory distress syndrome.

85. Which of the following is *not* a purpose of a conventional ventilator when used in tandem with HFJV?

   A. Its sigh breaths stimulate production of surfactant.

   B. Its sigh breaths prevent microatelectasis.

   C. It provides pressure support ventilation.

   D. It provides a continuous gas flow for entrainment by HFJV.

86. What is the major hazard of HFJV due to the impact of high-pressure gas on the wall of the airways?

_____

_____

87. To minimize the impact of high-pressure gas on the wall of the airways, HFJV should only be delivered through a special catheter that exits _____ (externally, internally) to the ET tube or via a special triple-lumen ET tube.

88. Besides necrotizing tracheobronchitis, name at least three other hazards of HFJV.

_____

_____

_____

89. Why is auscultation of breath sounds and heart sounds difficult during high frequency jet ventilation?

_____

_____

90. In place of auscultation, patient assessment during HFJV may be based on other clinical signs. Decreased lung compliance or pneumothoraces are observed by a(n) _____ (increase, decrease) in chest wall vibration, _____ (hypercapnia, hypocapnia), and _____ (hyperoxia, hypoxemia).

91. During HFJV, a(n) _____ (increase, decrease) in chest wall vibration and a(n) _____ (increase, decrease) in $PaCO_2$, without a drop in PaO_2, may indicate airway obstruction or malposition of the ET tube.

92. Tension pneumothoraces in the neonates may be detected by _____ of the chest when chest radiograph is not readily available.

93. High frequency oscillatory ventilation (HFOV) utilizes the highest of frequencies, usually in the range of _____ to _____/min or _____ to _____ Hz.

94. A unique feature of the high frequency oscillatory ventilator is that it produces extremely rapid _____ cycles.

    A. inspiratory

    B. expiratory

    C. inspiratory and expiratory

    D. spontaneous breathing

95. Modern high frequency oscillatory ventilators may be provided with simple traditional ET tubes and are not used in tandem with conventional ventilators. _____ (TRUE/FALSE)

96. HFOV should be considered when _____ (oxygen hood, N-CPAP, mechanical ventilation, BiPAP) fails to provide adequate ventilation or oxygenation to neonates of all birth weights and gestational ages.

97. HFOV is also effective in stabilizing neonates with congenital diaphragmatic hernia, air leak, pulmonary hypoplasia. _____ (TRUE/FALSE)

98. A rapidly increasing oxygen requirement may be present when the oxygen index is _____ (greater than 10, less than 10).

99. The radiographic signs of hyaline membrane disease (HMD) include _____ (diffuse, localized) homogeneous lung disease _____ (with, without) evidence of air trapping.

100. HFOV _____ (enhances, prevents) the release of inflammatory chemical mediators in the lung, resulting in fewer _____ (cardiovascular complications, lung injuries) than are seen with conventional ventilation.

101. When HFOV is used in conjunction with _____ replacement therapy soon after birth, the incidence and severity of bronchopulmonary dysplasia may be reduced.

102. The ability of HFOV to oxygenate the blood is _____ (better than, equally effective as, not as good as) other methods of ventilation. Use of _____ (high, low) levels of PEEP is generally done.

103. During HFJV and HFOV, signs of pallor, cyanosis, _____ (tachycardia, bradycardia), _____ (hypertension, hypotension), and increased respiratory effort are indicative of a worsening patient status.

104. The mean airway pressure (mPaw) affects mostly the _____ (airway pressure, acid-base balance, oxygenation status) of the infant.

105. The mean airway pressure (mPaw) during HFOV is primarily determined by the _____ (bias flow, frequency, power setting).

106. For infants with diffuse alveolar disease such as HMD, the mPaw during HFOV should be maintained at a level that is _____ (1 to 2, 3 to 4, 5 to 6, 7 to 8) cm H_2O higher than the mPaw recorder during conventional ventilation.

107. The bias flow during HFOV ranges from _____ (5 to 10, 10 to 15, 15 to 20) L/min for infants less than 2000 g and _____ (20, 40, 60) L/min for those greater than 2000 g.

108. The power setting of HFOV determines all of the following parameters *except*:

    A. tidal volume.

    B. inspiratory time %.

    C. degree of ventilation.

    D. amplitude of oscillation.

109. When the power setting is changed during HFOV, the mPaw is self-adjusted to an appropriate level. _____ (TRUE/FALSE)

110. The initial frequency setting for HFOV ranges from _____ (2 to 7, 8 to 15, 16 to 20) Hz.

111. During HFOV, a _____ (higher, lower) frequency provides a larger tidal volume during HFOV.

112. Chest wiggle is determined by observable chest movement down to the _____ (7th, 8th, 9th) ribs or umbilicus during HFOV.

OTHER METHODS OF VENTILATION

113. Dual control refers to a breath type that combines the useful features of two modes of ventilation. Name these two modes.

    _____

    _____

114. With the *Machine Volume* mode in the AVEA ventilator, the clinician sets a target _____ (tidal volume, peak inspiratory pressure) and inspiratory time, and the ventilator delivers the _____ (tidal volume, peak inspiratory pressure) using variable _____ (pressure, flow) to meet the patient's resistance, compliance, and flow demands.

115. With the *Volume Guarantee* mode in the Babylog 8000 plus ventilator, the clinician sets the:

    A. tidal volume.

    B. maximal peak inspiratory pressure.

    C. inspiratory time.

    D. A and B only.

116. Immediately before delivery of tidal volume breaths by the Babalog 8000 plus, the ventilator monitors the preceding _____ (inspiratory pressure, expired tidal volume) and makes breath-by-breath adjustments of the _____ (inspiratory time, inspiratory pressure, expired tidal volume) to deliver the set tidal volume.

117. Perfluorochemicals (PFC) are _____ (gases, liquids, powders) that have been used successfully to support _____ (perfusion, respiration) at very _____ (high, low) pulmonary _____ (blood pressure, inflation pressure).

EXTRACORPOREAL MEMBRANE OXYGENATION (ECMO)

118. Extracorporeal membrane oxygenation (ECMO) is a technique to oxygenate the blood _____ (by a ventilator, by blood transfusion, outside the body).

119. ECMO is not recommended for infants of less than _____ weeks of gestational age, weighing less than _____ g, having evidence of _____ hemorrhage.

120. ECMO is contraindicated when mechanical ventilation has been used for more than _____ weeks prior to the initiation of ECMO. This is because of an increased incidence of _____ (pulmonary hypertension, congestive heart failure, chronic lung disease), which ECMO cannot reverse.

121. Potential candidates for ECMO may include neonates with persistent pulmonary hypertension of the newborn (PPHN), meconium aspiration syndrome (MAS), sepsis, and congenital diaphragmatic hernia. _____ (TRUE/FALSE)

122. ECMO therapy is reserved for candidates with extremely high mortality rate (80% or greater) under conventional mechanical ventilation strategies. Which of the following methods is not used to predict mortality?

    A. Alveolar-arterial oxygen pressure gradient [$P(A-a)O_2$]

    B. Oxygen index

    C. Oxygen consumption and cardiac output

    D. PaO_2 or pH measurements

123. A $P(A-a)O_2$ value of _____ to _____ mm Hg at 100% F_IO_2 for 4 to 12 hours is indicative for ECMO therapy since it is consistent with _____ (mild, moderate, severe) hypoxemia.

124. A neonate has the following umbilical arterial blood gases: pH = 7. 34, $PaCO_2$ = 45 mm Hg, PaO_2 = 68 mm Hg, F_IO_2 = 100%. What is the $P(A-a)O_2$ if the barometric pressure is 748 mm Hg?

    A. 588 mm Hg

    B. 635 mm Hg

    C. 680 mm Hg

    D. 703 mm Hg

125. Infants with an oxygen index of _____ to _____ for 30 minutes to 6 hours are inclusive for ECMO therapy because this condition reflects _____ (high, low) airway pressures in conjunction with hypoxemia.

126. An infant has the following measurements: mean airway pressure = 25 cm H_2O, PaO_2 = 45 mm Hg at an F_IO_2 of 60%. What is the calculated oxygen index?

    A. 15

    B. 33

    C. 67

    D. 82

127. A third criterion for ECMO therapy is the presence of a PaO_2 of _____ to _____ mm Hg for 2 to 12 hours or a pH of less than _____ for 2 hours with _____ (hypertension, hypotension).

128. In the venoarterial route, blood is drawn from the _____ (left, right) atrium via the _____ (external, internal) jugular vein. The oxygenated blood is returned to the _____ (left atrium, aortic arch) via the right common _____ (brachial, femoral, carotid) artery.

129. Explain how the venoarterial ECMO supports the cardiac function of the patient.

_____

_____

130. With the venovenous route for ECMO, blood is removed from the _____ (left, right) atrium via the _____ (left, right) internal jugular vein. The oxygenated blood is returned to the _____ (aortic arch, right atrium, left atrium) through a catheter inserted via the _____ (femoral artery, femoral vein).

131. The venovenous method for ECMO oxygenates the blood, and it also supports a patient's cardiac output. _____ (TRUE/FALSE)

132. List at least three *pulmonary* complications of ECMO.

_____

_____

_____

133. What are the two major *cardiovascular* complications of ECMO?

_____

_____

134. _____ (Polycythemia, Anemia), _____ (leukocytosis, leukopenia), and _____ (thrombocytosis, thrombocytopenia) are possible hematologic complications of ECMO. This is caused by the _____ (creation, consumption) of blood components by the membrane oxygenator.

CHAPTER 18

Mechanical Ventilation in Nontraditional Settings

MECHANICAL VENTILATION AT HOME

1. Advantages of providing mechanical ventilation in the patient's home include all of the following *except*:

   A. extension and enhancement of quality of life.

   B. improvement of patient's physical and physiologic functions.

   C. reduction of cost for mechanical ventilation.

   D. reduction of stress level of family members.

2. A patient being mechanically ventilated at home is more likely to become _____ (more active, indifferent, more passive) in the weaning or rehabilitation process.

3. Interactions with family members and friends at home will enhance the patient's _____ (physical, spiritual, psychologic, medical) well-being and quality of life.

4. Since the cost savings of providing mechanical ventilation at home can be drastic, it should be the primary consideration in sending a patient from the hospital to home. _____ (TRUE/FALSE)

5. The most important ingredient of a successful home ventilator care program is probably the:

   A. financial resources of the patient.

   B. dedication and commitment of home care team members.

   C. insurance policy of the patient.

   D. availability of state-of-the-art equipment.

6. What are the four questions that may be helpful in assessing the indications for providing mechanical ventilation at home?

   _____

   _____

   _____

   _____

7 to 10. Many different diseases may be managed with home mechanical ventilation. Match the pulmonary problems with the respective clinical courses. Use each answer only *once*.

PULMONARY PROBLEM	CLINICAL COURSE
7. _____ Chronic obstructive pulmonary disease (COPD)	A. Inefficient ventilatory muscle, atelectasis, pneumonia
8. _____ Restrictive lung disease	B. Apnea, chronic hypoventilation, atelectasis, pneumonia
9. _____ Ventilatory muscle dysfunction	C. Reduction of lung volumes and capacities, deadspace ventilation, muscle fatigue
10. _____ Central hypoventilation syndrome	D. Airflow obstruction, excessively high compliance, air trapping, acute exacerbation

11. Patients with a stable COPD condition typically have blood gases showing _____ (acute, chronic) ventilatory failure or _____ (compensated, uncompensated) respiratory acidosis.

12. When COPD patients develop ventilatory failure or oxygenation failure, blood gases usually show _____ (acute, chronic) ventilatory failure superimposed on _____ (acute, chronic) ventilatory failure.

13. Define acute exacerbation of COPD.

_____

_____

_____

14. Which of the following blood gas reports best illustrates acute exacerbation of COPD?

   A. pH = 7.36, $PaCO_2$ = 55 mm Hg, PaO_2 = 50 mm Hg, HCO_3^- = 30 mEq/L

   B. pH = 7.38, $PaCO_2$ = 46 mm Hg, PaO_2 = 75 mm Hg, HCO_3^- = 26 mEq/L

   C. pH = 7.27, $PaCO_2$ = 74 mm Hg, PaO_2 = 43 mm Hg, HCO_3^- = 33 mEq/L

   D. pH = 7.20, $PaCO_2$ = 42 mm Hg, PaO_2 = 43 mm Hg, HCO_3^- = 16 mEq/L

15. Why are COPD patients more difficult to wean from mechanical ventilation than non-COPD patients?

_____

_____

16. The primary problem of restrictive lung disease is the reduction of _____ (airflow, lung volumes). Patients with restrictive lung disease usually assume a _____ (rapid and shallow, slow and deep) breathing pattern.

17. The ratio of deadspace/tidal volume is _____ (increased, decreased) during rapid shallow breathing. This occurs because the anatomic deadspace volume is _____ (increased, stable, decreased) while the tidal volume is decreased.

18. The work of breathing in restrictive lung diseases is _____ (higher, lower) than normal because of the _____ (high, low) lung compliance characteristic.

19. In the early stage, patients with uncomplicated ventilatory muscle dysfunction usually have _____ (healthy, unhealthy) lungs.

20. Under what conditions do patients with restrictive lung disorder need mechanical ventilation?

_____

_____

_____

21. A patient who was in an accident sustained severe spinal cord injuries at the cervical 2 (C-2) level. If the injuries impair the spinal function at this level, this patient is most likely a candidate for long-term:

    A. aerosol therapy.

    B. nasal CPAP therapy.

    C. oxygen therapy.

    D. mechanical ventilation.

22. Regardless of the etiology, patients with central hypoventilation syndrome often require around-the-clock mechanical ventilation. _____ (TRUE/FALSE)

23. What are the primary pulmonary problems of persistent hypoventilation due to dysfunction of the autonomic control of breathing?

_____

_____

24. What are the two clinical criteria that preclude a hospitalized patient from receiving mechanical ventilation at home?

_____

_____

25. In addition to the clinical criteria for discharge planning, the decision to send the patient home should also be based on the desires of the:

    A. physician.

    B. patient.

    C. insurance carrier.

    D. hospital administrator.

26. Potential candidates for home ventilator care should be told about the potential _____ (advantages, disadvantages, advantages and disadvantages) of leaving the hospital and entering a home care environment.

27. List two *advantages* gained by a ventilator-dependent patient leaving the hospital and entering a home care environment.

_____

_____

28. List two *disadvantages* experienced by a ventilator-dependent patient leaving the hospital and entering a home care environment.

_____

_____

29. Explain why the discussions concerning home ventilator care should not take place when the patient is hypoxic, confused, or under emotional distress.

_____

_____

30. Why is it essential that the desires of the family members be considered before making plans for home mechanical ventilation?

_____

_____

31. What are the two major expenses of home ventilator care?

_____

_____

32. Home ventilator care can be justified from a financial standpoint when its total cost is _____ (higher than, same as, lower than) the cost of comparable hospital care.

33. Adequate space for the ventilator, special bed, wheelchair, oxygen units, and supplies are some concerns that are related to the _____ (physical resources, technical support, emotional support) of home ventilator care.

34. If the patient does not have adequate spontaneous ventilation for an extended period of time, _____ are the equipment of choice for home mechanical ventilation.

    A. chest cuirass and pneumobelt

    B. raincoat and wrap

    C. rocking bed and diaphragmatic pacing

    D. positive pressure or negative pressure ventilators

35. Under what condition is a backup ventilator necessary in a home care setting?

_____

_____

36. One negative-pressure ventilation device that resembles a shell fitting over the patient's chest wall is called a _____ (chest cuirass, raincoat or wrap, pneumobelt, rocking bed).

37. The _____ is another negative-pressure ventilation device that is an airtight jacket capable of sealing the arms, hips, and neck.

38. Explain how the pneumobelt provides ventilation.

_____

_____

39. The rocking bed relies on _____ (positive pressure, negative pressure, motion) to displace the abdominal contents, to facilitate diaphragmatic motion and ventilation.

40. Diaphragmatic pacing _____ (provides, augments) ventilation by stimulation of the thoracic _____ (arteries, veins, phrenic nerves).

41. Why should a home care ventilator be extremely dependable?

_____

_____

42. Why should a home care ventilator be simple to operate?

_____

_____

43. What are two advantages of ventilators with built-in rechargeable battery packs?

_____

_____

MECHANICAL VENTILATION IN MASS CASUALTY INCIDENTS

44. Mass casualty refers to a large number of _____ (injured, severely injured) or deaths that exceeds a timely response from regional support centers.

45. Tsunami, earthquakes, and pandemics are three examples of _____ (natural, man-made) mass casualty incidents.

46. Wars and terrorism are two examples of _____ (natural, man-made) mass casualty incidents.

47. Victims who suffer primary blast injury to the lungs typically require mechanical ventilation, fluid management, and supportive care. _____ (TRUE/FALSE)

48. Nerve agents used in war or terrorism acts are acetylcholinesterase _____ (enhancers, inhibitors) that lead to an accumulation of acetylcholine at the muscarinic and nicotinic receptors throughout the body. A _____ (sudden surge, gradual buildup) of acetylcholine may quickly induce loss of consciousness, seizures, flaccid paralysis, and apnea.

49. Compared to the Spanish Flu (influenza A/H1N1) pandemic that caused 50 to 100 million deaths worldwide, the H1N1 outbreaks in 2009 showed a _____ (higher, lower) mortality rate, due to a better knowledge base of the disease and quick implementation of isolation procedures.

50. Among those patients with confirmed cases during the H1N5 outbreaks in 2009, many developed acute lung injury or acute respiratory distress syndrome and required _____ (oxygen therapy, noninvasive positive pressure ventilation, mechanical ventilation).

51. Based on a 2005 estimate by the U.S. Department of Health and Human Services, more than _____ (6,000, 60,000, 600,000) ventilators would be required for a 1958/68-like pandemic.

52. _____ (Classification, Sort, Triage) is a process using predetermined criteria to assign individuals from a large pool of people for grouping and making decisions.

53. In the U.S. and most countries, triage puts a high priority of care on those _____ (mildly, severely) ill individuals who are most likely to survive.

54. START is a simple triage and rapid-treatment algorithm suitable for use by _____ (hospital health care providers, first-responders).

55. START is based on two parameters: respirations and perfusion. _____ (TRUE/FALSE)

56. START and JumpSTART are triage systems for mass casualty incidents performed _____ (before, after) admission to a health care facility.

57. JumpSTART is a triage system for _____ (adults, children).

58. SALT is a triage system done _____ (prehospitalization, during hospitalization).

59. SALT stands for:

    A. Save, Assign, Lift to aircraft, Treatment/Transport.

    B. Sort, Assign, Leave for hospital, Treatment.

    C. Sort, Assess, Life-saving interventions, Treatment/Transport.

    D. Save, Assess, Lift to aircraft, Transport.

60. LSI in SALT stands for life-saving intervention. _____ (TRUE/FALSE)

61. Life-saving intervention in SALT incorporates: control major hemorrhage, open airway, and chest compression. _____ (TRUE/FALSE)

62. SOFA stands for Severe Organ Failure Assessment. _____ (TRUE/FALSE)

63. The Sequential Organ Failure Assessment (SOFA) is a triage system done _____ (prehospitalization, during hospitalization).

64. SOFA uses _____ (4, 6, 8) criteria to predict the outcomes of critically ill patients in the hospital.

65. List the SOFA criteria.

_____

_____

_____

66. The parameters used in the SOFA scoring system are related to oxygenation, blood clotting, liver function, blood pressure, neurologic function, and kidney function. _____ (TRUE/FALSE).

67. A high SOFA score (e.g., ≥11) calls for _____ (highest priority of critical care, intermediate critical care, palliation care).

68. A high SOFA score (e.g., ≥11) correlates with a mortality rate of _____ (10%, 50%, 95%).

69. A SOFA score from _____ (10 to 8, 6 to 2) calls for the highest priority of critical care.

70. In 2006, the Strategic National Stockpile (SNS) program owned and maintained approximately _____ (600, 6,000, 15,000, 50,000) mechanical ventilators for distribution to states affected by mass casualty.

71. Disadvantages of a national Strategic National Stockpile (SNS) program include the potential lack of experience and trouble-shooting skills by clinicians with the _____ (common, brand-specific) ventilators in the stockpile.

72. In the stockpile of mechanical ventilators, the LTV 1200 (CareFusion) and Newport HT50 portable ventilators are being replaced by the LP-10 and Uni-Vent Eagle 754. _____ (TRUE/FALSE)

73. For individuals meeting the exclusion criteria, they _____ (would, would not) be placed on a ventilator should the number of ventilators fail to meet the surge in demand.

74. The exclusion criteria used by the New York State Department of Health (NYS DOH) are based on _____ (subjective, objective) clinical conditions and _____ (rely, do not rely) on ethical or quality-of-life issues.

75. The exclusion criteria used by the NYS DOH focus on 3 areas: a person's history of cardiac arrest, presence of metastatic malignancy, and organ failure. _____ (TRUE/FALSE)

76. List the 5 organs or systems that are evaluated during the organ-failure assessment in the exclusion criteria used by the NYS DOH.

_____

_____

_____

_____

_____

77. An effective emergency preparedness program _____ (must, may not) include the training exercise and evaluation components.

MECHANICAL VENTILATION IN HYPERBARIC CONDITIONS

78. List 4 conditions that hyperbaric oxygen (HBO) may be useful as a treatment modality.

_____

_____

_____

_____

79. At an F_IO_2 of 21%, the normal oxygen content is 20 vol% and the plasma carries about _____ (0.3 vol%, 3 vol%) of the total oxygen content.

80. At one atmospheric pressure (760 mm Hg at sea level) and an F_IO_2 of 100%, the PaO_2 is about 673 mm Hg and the calculated dissolved oxygen is about _____ (0.8 vol%, 2 vol%, 4.5 vol%).

81. At three (3) atmospheric pressures and an F_IO_2 of 100%, the calculated dissolved oxygen is about _____ (2.4 vol%, 6 vol%, 13.5 vol%).

82. Since tissues require a minimum of 6 ml of oxygen per liter of blood flow to maintain normal metabolism, an F_IO_2 of 100% at three (3) atmospheric pressures _____ (would, would not) meet this demand.

83. Decompression sickness occurs when a diver ascends to the water surface too _____ (rapidly, slowly). Rapid decompression of pressure causes the dissolved gases in blood to form gas bubbles which can migrate to the _____ (lungs, joints and tissues).

84. Decompression sickness can also occur when a person: (choose A or B)

    A. descends rapidly from high altitude over 18,000 ft to low altitude.

    B. ascends rapidly from low altitude to high altitude over 18,000 ft.

85. Treatment for decompression sickness from diving or high mountain adventure includes recompression _____ (gradually, rapidly) in a hyperbaric chamber followed by _____ (gradual, rapid) decompression.

86. In mild-to-moderate carbon monoxide poisoning, the patient may be treated with 100% inspired oxygen until the carboxyhemoglobin level is less than _____ (1%, 5%, 10%).

87. In severe carbon monoxide poisoning, hyperbaric oxygen (HBO) is useful to prevent tissue hypoxia, because HBO increases the oxygen content by increasing the amount of oxygen _____ (combined with hemoglobin, dissolved in plasma).

88. _____ (Aerobic, Anaerobic) infections (e.g., _Clostridium perfringens_) respond to hyperbaric oxygen in some cases because an oxygen-enriched environment hinders the growth of _____ (aerobic, anaerobic) pathogens.

89. For patients requiring an endotracheal tube in the hyperbaric chamber, _____ (water, saline, air) is used to fill the cuff of the endotracheal tube. This is done to prevent overdistension and rupture of the cuff during _____ (compression, decompression).

90. Pressure-controlled ventilation (PCV) is preferred when mechanical ventilation is required in a multiplace hyperbaric chamber, because this mode of ventilation delivers a more stable tidal volume during _____ (compression, decompression, compression and decompression).

91. Volume-controlled ventilation (VCV) requires frequent adjustments of the _____ (peak inspiratory pressure, tidal volume) during compression and decompression.

92. Most ventilators designed for hyperbaric application can withstand pressure as high as _____ (4, 6, 8) times the atmospheric pressure.

93. Boyle's Law ($V_1 \times P_1 = V_2 \times P_2$) shows the _____ (direct, inverse) relationship between pressure and volume.

94. In volume-controlled ventilation under hyperbaric conditions, the delivered tidal volume is _____ (more, less) than the set tidal volume. This is because a higher pressure causes _____ (more, less) compression to the volume, resulting in a _____ (larger, smaller) delivered volume.

95. As the pressure increases in the multiplace hyperbaric chamber, the set tidal volume should be _____ (increased, decreased) to compensate for the effects of gas compression.

96. In mechanical ventilation, the expired volume is usually _____ (greater than, about the same as) the delivered volume.

97. The expired tidal volume may be monitored by a _____ (peak flow meter, mechanical respirometer) during gas compression and decompression.

98. The tidal volume setting can be adjusted based on the _____ (expired tidal volume, peak inspiratory pressure).

99. During hyperbaric oxygen therapy, the electrocardiogram (ECG) signals _____ (remain inside, are transferred outside) the hyperbaric chamber for monitoring.

100. Use of a pulse oximeter in the hyperbaric chamber is limited to the pulse rate only, because HBO usually results in _____ (90%, 100%) oxygen saturation for patients without cardiovascular deficits.

101. To prevent fire hazards, a(n) _____ (electronic, manual) blood pressure measuring device should be used in the hyperbaric chamber.

102. Cardiac output, intracranial pressure, and blood gas analysis are some invasive procedures that can be performed safely under hyperbaric conditions. _____ (TRUE/FALSE)

103. Defibrillation _____ (should not, may) be performed under hyperbaric conditions.

104. Most implanted cardiac pacemakers can be used safely in the hyperbaric chamber for pressures below _____ (3, 6) atmospheres.

MECHANICAL VENTILATION IN HYPOBARIC CONDITIONS

105. At 8,000 ft above sea level, the barometric pressure (P_B) is _____ (776 mm Hg, 564 mm Hg) and the calculated P_AO_2 at this altitude is _____ (59 mm Hg, 39 mm Hg). An acute drop in the P_B and P_AO_2 are the primary reasons for _____ (decompression, high-altitude) illness experienced by unacclimatized persons.

106. Upon arrival at Mount Elbert, Colorado (altitude 14,433 ft above sea level), a person complains of sudden headache, nausea, insomnia, and fatigue. The most likely diagnosis is _____ (compression sickness, decompression sickness, acute mountain sickness).

107. High-altitude cerebral edema is related to _____ (vasoconstriction, vasodilatation) of cerebral vessels, overperfusion, and inadequate volume buffering by cerebrospinal fluid.

108. The treatment for acute mountain sickness includes descent to a lower altitude, use of supplemental oxygen, acetazolamide (Diamox), and dexamethasone. _____ (TRUE/FALSE)

109. High-altitude pulmonary edema is primarily _____ (cardiogenic, noncardiogenic) in origin, but it is associated with pulmonary hypertension and elevated capillary pressure.

110. Decreased endurance, dry cough, pink or bloody sputum, resting tachycardia, and tachypnea are signs of high-altitude _____ (cerebral edema, pulmonary edema).

111. The incidence of acute mountain sickness and high-altitude pulmonary edema is related to the rate of _____ (descent to low altitude, ascent to high altitude) and the altitude reached.

112. The treatment for high-altitude _____ (cerebral edema, pulmonary edema) includes descent to lower altitude, supplemental oxygen, and portable hyperbaric chamber.

113. Nifedipine, a _____ (potassium, calcium) channel blocker, may be used when descent is not possible or medical equipment and supplies are not available.

114. Airplanes can fly more efficiently at higher altitudes because the air becomes _____ (more, less) dense and the airflow resistance to the airplane is _____ (higher, lower).

115. Most commercial airplanes travel at a cruising altitude between 25,000 ft and 40,000 ft, and the airplane cabin pressure altitude ranges from _____ (0 ft to 1,000 ft, 2,000 ft to 4,000 ft, 5,000 ft to 8,000 ft).

116. For the safety and comfort of the passengers inside the commercial airplane, most airplanes are pressurized to a cabin pressure altitude of _____ (1,000 ft, 4,000 ft, 8,000 ft). At this altitude, a P_AO_2 of _____ (126 mm Hg, 100 mm Hg, 59 mm Hg, 37 mm Hg) can lead to high-altitude hypoxia.

117. As a general guideline, supplemental oxygen should be used when a person's pulse oximetry measurement is _____ (3%, 5%, 7%, 10%) below the normal value for home altitude.

118. At 10,000 ft cabin pressure altitude, individuals have a tolerated SpO_2 range from _____ (83 to 87%, 88% to 93%, 93 to 98%).

119. During mechanical ventilation at high altitudes, the measured tidal volume and peak flow _____ (increase, decrease) as the barometric pressures decrease (from low altitude to high altitude).

120. The gas _____ (expands, contracts) during ascent. For mechanically ventilated patients, this _____ (increasing, decreasing) tidal volume during ascent can cause hyperinflation and become potentially harmful.

121. During mechanical ventilation at a high altitude, _____ (volume-, pressure-) compensated ventilators tend to deliver stable tidal volume, peak inspiratory flow, peak proximal airway pressure, and minute ventilation.

122. Capability, battery life, weight, dimensions, and alarms are some important features of a _____ (stationary, portable) ventilator.

123. All portable ventilators are capable of using battery and wall outlet electrical sources. _____ (TRUE/FALSE)

124. Prior to making travel plans for a ventilator-dependent person, the traveler should prepare all of the following *except*:

    A. obtain physician's written permission to travel with a portable ventilator.

    B. purchase an extra ticket for a seat adjacent to the traveler.

    C. locate a destination home care company that provides portable ventilators.

    D. gather adequate battery packs and supplies for the portable ventilator.

125. Commercial airlines _____ (are, are not) required by the FAA to provide electrical connection in the plane for portable ventilators or oxygen concentrators.

126. A(n) _____ (airport attendant, personal traveling companion) may be required if the traveler needs a higher level of service and medical support.

127. When an airplane takes off and ascends to a higher altitude, a lower barometric pressure causes the gas density to _____ (increase, decrease) and the gas volume (tidal volume) to _____ (increase, decrease).

128. During airplane *ascent* with a non-pressure-compensated ventilator, the set tidal volume should be _____ (increased, decreased) to prevent _____ (inadequate tidal volume, hyperinflation).

129. During airplane *descent* with a non-pressure-compensated ventilator, the set tidal volume should be _____ (increased, decreased) to prevent _____ (inadequate tidal volume, hyperinflation).

130. It is estimated that the tidal volume can be *reduced* by 3% per 1,000 ft of _____ (ascent, descent) or *increased* by 3% per 1,000 ft of _____ (ascent, descent).

131. High-altitude _____ (hypercapnia, hypoxia) can be minimized by using a portable oxygen concentrator.

132. The airlines in the U.S. _____ (are, are not) required to provide supplemental oxygen during flights.

133. Weight and duration of battery life are two important elements of a _____ (stationary, portable) oxygen concentrator.

134. Commercial airlines _____ (are, are not) required to provide direct-current electricity for the portable oxygen concentrator.

NOTES

NOTES

NOTES

NOTES

NOTES

NOTES

NOTES

NOTES